Medical Insights

From Classroom to Patient

Morton A. Diamond, MD, FACP, FACC, FAHA
Medical Director and Professor
Physician Assistant Program
Nova Southeastern University
Fort Lauderdale, Florida

D1529248

JONES AND BARTLETT PUBLISHERS
Sudbury, Massachusetts
BOSTON   TORONTO   LONDON   SINGAPORE

World Headquarters

Jones and Bartlett Publishers	Jones and Bartlett Publishers	Jones and Bartlett Publishers
40 Tall Pine Drive	Canada	International
Sudbury, MA 01776	6339 Ormindale Way	Barb House, Barb Mews
978-443-5000	Mississauga, Ontario L5V 1J2	London W6 7PA
info@jbpub.com	Canada	UK
www.jbpub.com		

Jones and Bartlett's books and products are available through most bookstores and online booksellers. To contact Jones and Bartlett Publishers directly, call 800-832-0034, fax 978-443-8000, or visit our website, www.jbpub.com.

Substantial discounts on bulk quantities of Jones and Bartlett's publications are available to corporations, professional associations, and other qualified organizations. For details and specific discount information, contact the special sales department at Jones and Bartlett via the above contact information or send an email to specialsales@jbpub.com.

The author, editor, and publisher have made every effort to provide accurate information. However, they are not responsible for errors, omissions, or for any outcomes related to the use of the contents of this book and take no responsibility for the use of the products and procedures described. Treatments and side effects described in this book may not be applicable to all people; likewise, some people may require a dose or experience a side effect that is not described herein. Drugs and medical devices are discussed that may have limited availability controlled by the Food and Drug Administration (FDA) for use only in a research study or clinical trial. Research, clinical practice, and government regulations often change the accepted standard in this field. When consideration is being given to use of any drug in the clinical setting, the health care provider or reader is responsible for determining FDA status of the drug, reading the package insert, and reviewing prescribing information for the most up-to-date recommendations on dose, precautions, and contraindications, and determining the appropriate usage for the product. This is especially important in the case of drugs that are new or seldom used.

Production Credits
Publisher: David Cella
Associate Editor: Maro Gartside
Editorial Assistant: Teresa Reilly
Production Director: Amy Rose
Senior Production Editor: Renée Sekerak
Marketing Manager: Grace Richards
Manufacturing and Inventory Control Supervisor: Amy Bacus
Cover and Title Page Design: Kristin E. Parker
Cover Image: Chalkboard, © Carolina K. Smith, M.D./ShutterStock, Inc.; Doctor and patient,
    © Iofoto/Dreamstime.com
Composition: Paw Print Media
Printing and Binding: Malloy Incorporated
Cover Printing: John Pow Company

Library of Congress Cataloging-in-Publication Data
Diamond, Morton A.
  Medical insights : from classroom to patient / by Morton A. Diamond.
      p. ; cm.
  Includes bibliographical references and index.
  ISBN-13: 978-0-7637-5284-2
  ISBN-10: 0-7637-5284-3
  1. Internal medicine—Handbooks, manuals, etc. I. Title.
  [DNLM: 1. Clinical Medicine—methods. WB 102 D537m 2010]
  RC55.D525 2010
  616—dc22
                          2009017814
6048

Printed in the United States of America
13 12 11 10 09   10 9 8 7 6 5 4 3 2 1

Dedication

To my wife, Louise, and to the memory of our parents, Ann and Paul Diamond and Frances and Irving Goldman.

Contents

Preface

Traditional textbooks are exhaustive in content. Yet, their *strength* is their *weakness*. In an effort to present the voluminous material in a logical fashion, the books are, most frequently, organized by functional systems, e.g., gastroenterology, cardiology, and endocrinology. It is unavoidable that presented information becomes fragmented and, therefore, difficult for the student to understand and retain. For example, ptosis, drooping of the eyelid, is presented in the following chapters in a medicine text: pulmonary (bronchogenic carcinoma), autoimmune diseases (myasthenia gravis), neurology (intracranial aneurysm), endocrinology (diabetes mellitus), infectious disease (Lyme disease), and diseases of unknown etiology (sarcoidosis).

This book is not a textbook. It is not designed to present voluminous information. Rather, it is a book designed to express a clinician's *approach to medical thinking in the diagnosis and management of the patient.* Voluminous and disjointed information is distilled into a more easily understood format.

Let us return to the earlier example, ptosis. In this book, the subject of ptosis is succinctly presented, in a clinically relevant and easy-to-understand manner. What are the 3 questions, all quickly answered on physical examination, that enable the clinician to quickly determine the cause of ptosis? Is the ptosis greater (or less) than 3 mm? What is the pupil size of the affected eye? Are the extraocular eye movements normal on the affected side?

Chapters are not organized by organ systems. Rather, their titles represent the thinking of the clinician. Chapter titles include:

- Medical Brevities
- The Most Important Word in Diagnosis: *And*
- MED1C and a Word on Drug Interactions
- Stop . . . and Think
- Always and Never

- Linkages
- The Smartest Answer to a Medical Question: "It Depends"
- Clinical Potpourri

The chapter titles express the theme of this book, to collate medical information in a clinically relevant and understandable format. Principles of therapy are emphasized. However, specific details in clinical pharmacology and disease treatment have been eschewed in order to avoid an expansive dimension to the book.

It would be most satisfying to me if the reader finds this book to be valuable in patient care and, at the same time, pleasurable reading.

About the Author

Morton A. Diamond, MD, FACP, FACC, FAHA, is a clinical cardiologist with nearly four decades' experience in the education of medical students, physician assistant students, and graduate physicians. Since 1994 he has been the full-time Medical Director of the Nova Southeastern University Physician Assistant Program in Fort Lauderdale, Florida.

Dr. Diamond has published many articles in peer-reviewed medical journals on the subjects of neurogenic orthostatic hypotension, ultrasound diagnosis of congenital heart disease, and valvular heart disease. He has written chapters in medical textbooks and is frequently invited to present lectures at state and national medical meetings.

Reviewers

Frank Ambriz, PA-C, MPAS
Chair
Physician Assistant Program
Assistant Professor
University of Texas–Pan American

Pam Harrison Chambers, MPH, PA-C
Physician Assistant Program Faculty
Des Moines University

Laura Delaney, PA-C
Physician Assistant Program Faculty
Des Moines University

Ahmad Hakemi, MD
Professor, Program Director
Central Michigan University

Kim Meyer, MPAS, PA-C
Program Director
Physician Assistant Program
Louisiana State University Health Sciences Center

Heidi B. Miller, PA-C, MPH
Director
Physician Assistant Program
Professor
Department of Medical Sciences
Rochester Institute of Technology

Frederick A. Schaller, DO, FACOI
Vice Dean and Professor
School of Osteopathic Medicine
Touro University–Nevada

Daniel T. Vetrosky, PA-C, PhD
Assistant Professor
Department of Physician Assistant Studies
University of South Alabama

Chapter 1

Medical Brevities

I n this chapter, I try to challenge your traditional thinking. The "brevities" are designed to inform, to suggest common denominators in seemingly varied medical conditions, and to provoke your thinking. You will never diagnose a disease if you do not think of it.

Brevity 1: A Deficiency in a Hematinic Agent May Cause Illness While the Blood Count Is Still Normal

Iron Deficiency

> Clinical vignette: A 36-year-old woman presents with a feeling of weakness, listlessness, and easy fatigability. The patient works part-time while raising her three children. Physical examination is normal. Hemoglobin is 12.0 g/dL, and the other blood elements are in the normal range. The clinician tells the patient, "Your physical examination is normal and your blood count is normal. I think you may well be depressed from your arduous workload. I suggest that you start this medication." A selective serotonin receptor inhibitor (SSRI) is prescribed.

The clinician must recognize that iron deficiency without anemia can cause the patient's symptoms. In this patient, a low serum ferritin (< 30 ng/mL) would document decreased iron stores while the hemoglobin, serum iron, and iron binding capacity are still in the normal range.

Iron deficiency occurs most often in the patient with increased blood loss, for example, from menstrual loss or from blood loss secondary to gastrointestinal bleeding, gross hematuria, trauma, or intravascular hemolysis (caused by loss of iron from hemoglobinuria and hemosiderinuria). Further, iron deficiency may occur with deficient oral intake or with impaired intestinal absorption of ingested iron. Impaired iron absorption is common in celiac disease and *Helicobacter pylori* gastritis and, less frequently, in autoimmune atrophic gastritis.

As the body deficiency in iron becomes more pronounced, the patient will develop the characteristic microcytic anemia.

Additionally, iron deficiency may cause other clinical illnesses. First, iron deficiency is one cause of restless leg syndrome (RLS). This disorder, twice as common in females than in males, is characterized by spontaneous, continuous leg movements associated with unpleasant paresthesias only when the patient is at rest. The symptoms, which are usually bilateral, are relieved by leg movement. Reduced levels of serum or spinal fluid ferritin are diagnostic of iron deficiency–related RLS. In these patients, the neurologic examination is normal. Other diseases and conditions known to be associated with RLS include end-stage renal disease, Parkinson's disease, venous insufficiency, and pregnancy. In pregnancy, the symptoms are most common in the third trimester; incidence drops quickly after delivery. Some patients with RLS have no recognized pathogenesis and are considered to be idiopathic or primary.

Second, iron deficiency may cause breath-holding syncope in children. This condition typically affects children who are 5 months to 6 years of age. (Ninety percent have the first episode before age 18 months.) The episodes are triggered by even mild emotional insults, anger, fear, or pain. The origin is considered to be a variant of vasovagal syncope. The syncopal episodes may be associated with a pallid or cyanotic skin hue. During syncopal episodes, the patient is limp and may exhibit seizure activity. Consultation with a pediatric neurologist is generally indicated to differentiate breath-holding syncope from a true seizure disorder.

Vitamin B$_{12}$ (Cobalamin) Deficiency

Clinical vignette: A 54-year-old man has progressive dementia of 7 months duration. Examination shows cognitive impairment. Propriception and vibratory sensation could not be adequately tested because of the patient's distractibility. Hemoglobin is 14.2 g/dL; other blood elements are normal. Red blood cell indices are normal.

The clinician must be aware that vitamin B$_{12}$ deficiency may cause severe neurologic manifestations while the hematocrit and red blood cell indices are normal. Intrinsic factor, produced in the gastric mucosa, is essential for cobalamin absorption in the distal ileum. Cobalamin deficiency is present in the autoimmune disease pernicious anemia because these patients have anti-intrinsic factor antibodies and, less commonly, anti-parietal cell antibodies. The anti-intrinsic factor antibodies prevent the vitamin absorption in the ileum. Other patients who do not have autoimmune disease may develop vitamin B_{12} deficiency. These include patients who have undergone gastrectomy and who do not produce intrinsic factor; patients who have inflammatory disease involving the terminal ileum and are unable to absorb cobalamin, for example, in Crohn's disease; patients with intestinal blind loop syndromes in which bacterial overgrowth competes for cobalamin; and those who follow a strict vegan diet without intake of dairy products, meat, and fish. Vitamin B_{12} is found only in food of animal origin.

Vitamin B_{12} deficiency causes a macrocytic and megaloblastic anemia as a result of impaired DNA formation in the premature erythrocyte. The vitamin deficiency impairs myelination of nerve fibers, resulting in neurologic deficits. The earliest neuropathic symptoms are paresthesias and ataxia. Early on, neurologic examination shows loss of vibratory sensation and proprioception due to degeneration of the posterior (dorsal) and lateral spinal columns. Higher nervous center impairment follows, with the patient exhibiting dementia or irritability.

Folic acid (folate) deficiency can produce the same megaloblastic anemia seen in cobalamin deficiency. However, folate deficiency does not cause neurologic impairment. Here is the key clinical element: In the patient who has vitamin B_{12} deficiency with anemia and neurologic deficit, the folate ingestion *will reverse the anemia but not the neuropathy*. To the question, How does vitamin B_{12} deficiency cause dementia and spinal cord degeneration while the blood count is normal, *the answer is that the cobalamin-deficient patient is ingesting adequate amounts of folate to prevent anemia*. (Dietary folate is found in green leafy vegetables in addition to multivitamin supplements.)

In the patient who has peripheral neuropathy or dementia while the hemoglobin and red blood cell indices are normal, vitamin B_{12} deficiency may be diagnosed by a low serum cobalamin level. If the cobalamin level is borderline low, an elevated serum methylmalonic acid level supports the diagnosis of vitamin B_{12} deficiency. If the vitamin B_{12} deficiency neuropathy is diagnosed at an early stage, it is reversible with cobalamin therapy.

You must remember:
1. Iron deficiency may cause significant symptoms of fatigue and lassitude while the hemoglobin level is still normal. A decreased level of serum ferritin is diagnostic of iron deficiency.
2. Vitamin B_{12} deficiency of any etiology may produce neurologic impairment (loss of proprioception and vibratory sensation) or dementia while the hemoglobin is normal. Ingestion of adequate folate will prevent the B_{12}-deficiency anemia but not the neuropathy.

Brevity 2: Not All Dementia Is Irreversible. The Clinician Must Always Look for a Treatable Cause of the Cognitive Disorder

Essentially irreversible causes of dementia include Alzheimer's disease, vascular (multi-infarct) dementia, Parkinson's disease, Huntington's chorea, and Lewy body dementia. Yet, there are potentially *treatable and reversible* causes of dementia. These patients may exhibit memory loss, impairment in calculation and judgment, and impaired problem solving. Patients who have the following disorders may improve with treatment:

- Depression
- Vitamin B_{12} (cobalamin) deficiency
- Medications
- Niacin deficiency
- Chronic subdural hematoma
- Normal pressure hydrocephalus (NPH)
- Hypothyroidism
- Bismuth poisoning
- Central nervous system tumors
- Whipple's disease

Depression often masquerades as dementia with memory loss and impaired judgment ("pseudodementia"). Appropriate treatment of the psychiatric disorder improves the patient's cognitive function. As noted earlier (see medical brevities 1), a neurologic manifestation of vitamin B_{12} deficiency may be dementia. If therapy with cobalamin is initiated early in its course, the dementia is reversible. Patients who have NPH will have dementia in addition to gait disorder and urinary incontinence. A ventricular shunting operative procedure can improve cognition in half of the patients operated on.

Particularly in the patient with impaired renal function, intake of bismuth, as in treatment of *Helicobacter pylori* gastritis, can cause confusion and dementia. Hypothyroidism can cause memory loss and depression, in addition to other classic manifestations, including weight gain, cold intolerance, and constipation. Serum thyroid stimulating hormone (TSH) levels are elevated in primary hypothyroidism, but are typically low in secondary hypothyroidism. Niacin deficiency, most commonly noted in the patient suffering from chronic alcohol abuse, can cause dementia. The patient may not exhibit the classic symptom triad of niacin deficiency in pellagra, namely, dermatitis, diarrhea, and dementia. Some patients with chronic subdural hematoma or primary brain tumor may present with dementia; in these patients motor signs may be subtle or absent. Many medicines may cause memory loss and cognitive dysfunction, including tranquilizers, sedatives, anticholinergic agents, and antidepressants. Whipple's disease is a rare bacterial illness. Patients commonly have arthralgia (or arthritis), abdominal pain, lymphadenopathy, fever, and dementia. Prolonged antibiotic therapy results in dramatic clinical improvement.

You must remember:
1. Though uncommon, the clinician must carefully search for a treatable cause in the patient who has dementia.

Brevity 3: Remember the "Acey-Ducey" Rule: In Paired Structures in the Body, *Recurrent* Involvement of One of the Pair Suggests a "Local" Disorder Whereas Involvement of Both Strongly Suggests Systemic Disease

Many years ago I was conscripted (physicians' draft) into the military and assigned to the Navy. I quickly learned of the Acey-Ducey clubs, the social clubs for first- and second-class petty (noncommissioned) officers. (No need to go into details of my social initiation to the clubs, including my introduction to the Salty Dog cocktail.) Thus, in my mind, *Acey* became "one" and *Ducey*, "two." Such is the provenance of my Acey-Ducey rule in medicine.

Clinical vignettes:

"Acey"
Over a 3-year-period, a 35-year-old man has had three attacks of renal colic related to kidney stones; all stones have been in the right kidney.

"Ducey"
A nurse at the hospital where I attended patients approached me one morning and anxiously told me that her son, a 20-year-old college student, just had a second episode of renal colic due to a kidney stone. I immediately asked her whether both attacks

involved one kidney, or whether both kidneys were involved. She answered that she did not know but would immediately inquire. A few minutes later, after speaking with her son, she informed me that the first stone was in the left kidney and the most recent attack involved the right kidney. I said to the nurse, "Ducey."

What is the important clinical difference?

"Acey"
A 47-year-old man has had three episodes of pneumonia in the past 4 months.

In each case, the infection was in the right lower lobe.

"Ducey"
A 33-year-old woman has had three episodes of pneumonia in the past 4 months. One episode of illness involved the left lower lobe, another involved the right middle lobe, and the most recent episode was pneumonia involving the left upper lobe.

What is the important clinical difference?

Two more vignettes:

"Ducey"
Three months ago, a 47-year-old man had carpal tunnel syndrome (CTS) involving his left wrist; he now has the disorder affecting his right wrist.

"Acey"
A 51-year-old woman who works as a secretary had CTS affecting her right wrist 2 years ago. With conservative therapy and nerve gliding exercises under the direction of an occupational therapist, she has had no recurrence.

What is the important clinical difference?

The Answer: First, consider that the kidneys, lungs, and wrists are paired structures in the body.

"Acey": Recurrent Involvement of One of the Paired Structures Suggests a "Local" Condition

Recurrent kidney stones involving *one* kidney suggest an underlying congenital anomaly or, perhaps, scarring from trauma or infection. Recurrent carpal tunnel involving *one* wrist suggests prior wrist trauma or Colles fracture or radiculopathy. Recurrent pneumonia in *one* lung (or *one* lobe) suggests an endobronchial lesion such as bronchogenic carcinoma, or, less often, a bron-cholith, or a local inflammatory disorder such as bronchiectasis.

"Ducey": Recurrent Involvement of Both of the Paired Structures Suggests a Systemic Disorder

Recurrent pneumonia that involves *both* lungs suggests a systemic disorder, most commonly, an immunocompromised state, such as HIV-AIDS or mul-tiple myeloma. In myeloma, impaired lymphocyte function and hypogamma-globulinemia predispose to recurrent pulmonary infections that can be present in any locus in the lungs ("Ping-Pong ball" pneumonia). HIV type 1 is a human retrovirus that infects lymphocytes and other cells that bear the CD4 surface protein. The resultant immune dysfunction results in recurrent pulmonary infections that involve both lungs.

Recurrent CTS that involves *both* wrists over a short time period (few months) suggests a systemic disorder. Approximately 30% of patients who have end-stage renal disease will have CTS. Commonly, patients who have hypothyroidism (7% of cases) and diabetes mellitus (6% of cases) have median nerve dysfunction. Seven percent of pregnant women have CTS; there is prompt resolution after delivery. Other systemic disorders that cause CTS are rheumatoid arthritis, acromegaly, and amyloidosis.

Recurrent kidney stones that involve *both* kidneys suggest a systemic dis-order such as hypercalcemia, idiopathic hypercalciuria, hyperuricemia, or cystinuria. Patients with gout have hyperuricemia and, therefore, are most susceptible to uric acid calculi in the kidneys. Cystinuria is a rare hered-itable disease with autosomal recessive transmission that should be consid-ered when a child has a renal calculus.

It is useful to separate hypercalcemia into two categories: hypercalcemia with low serum phosphate, and hypercalcemia with normal serum phosphate.

In the patient who has *hypercalcemia with a low serum phosphate*, think first of primary hyperparathyroidism, most commonly resulting from a soli-tary parathyroid adenoma (80% of cases) and, in the remaining 20% of cases, hyperplasia of the gland. Remember that primary hyperparathyroidism may, in selected patients, be part of a multiple endocrine neoplasia (MEN) syn-drome. Lithium therapy may result in increased serum parathyroid hormone secretion with similar serum chemical abnormalities.

Hypercalcemia in malignancy may be caused by three mechanisms. First is nonmetastatic tumor secretion of parathyroid-related protein resulting in hypercalcemia with low serum phosphate. T-cell lymphoma and B-cell non-Hodgkin's lymphoma are examples.

In contrast, *hypercalcemia may occur in association with a normal serum phosphate*. Examples include prolonged immobilization, myeloma, milk alkali syndrome, hyperthyroidism, thiazide diuretic therapy, malignancy, and sarcoidosis. Hypercalcemia occurs in 5% of sarcoidosis patients, but hypercalciuria is noted in 20%.

The other two mechanisms of malignancy-induced hypercalcemia include osteolytic metastases, most commonly resulting from breast and non-small cell lung cancer, and tumor production of calcitriol. Hodgkin's disease and, less commonly, non-Hodgkin's lymphoma are tumors that may produce calcitriol. In the body, vitamin D is activated to calcitriol, which increases intestinal absorption of calcium, increases parathyroid hormone bone resorption, and reduces urinary calcium and phosphate excretion. As a result, malignant disease related to these two mechanisms produces hypercalcemia with a normal serum phosphate concentration.

Milk alkali syndrome was common years ago when ingestion of milk and cream, in addition to bicarbonate compounds, was the mainstay of ulcer therapy. The syndrome now occurs in a different patient population. Patients now take calcium carbonate in the prevention or treatment of ostoporosis and, additionally, as part of a therapeutic program in eradication of *Helicobacter pylori* gastritis or ulcer. Milk alkali syndrome is characterized by hypercalcemia, elevated plasma bicarbonate, and azotemia. The serum phosphate level is most frequently normal, but may be slightly elevated in some patients.

You must remember the Acey-Ducey rule:
1. Think of paired structures in the body.
2. Recurrent involvement of one of the pair points toward a "local" disorder.
3. Recurrent involvement of both structures suggests systemic disease.

Brevity 4: Young Adults Can Suffer Acute Stroke. In These Patients, You Must Consider Patent Foramen Ovale, Factor V Leiden Mutation, and Antiphospholipid Antibody Syndrome as Causative Factors

Clinical vignette: I received an urgent phone call from one of my former medical students. With great anxiety, she stated that she was in a hospital emergency department with her 28-year-old firefighter husband who just spontaneously recovered from a

30-minute episode of weakness in his right arm and right leg. "What could it be?" she urgently inquired.

I first asked about his pulse. She responded that the pulse was normal in rate and was perfectly regular in rhythm. Immediately, it did not appear to be a cerebral embolus from a dislodged left atrial clot related to atrial fibrillation (AF). I then quickly probed about his general health. Her response was that he was robustly well.

Of course, I suggested immediate consultation, but volunteered that the three most likely causes, in descending order of frequency, were paradoxical embolus in a patent foramen ovale (PFO), antiphospholipid antibody syndrome (APS), or Factor V Leiden mutation. (One week later, he underwent percutaneous device closure of a PFO. After an appropriate period of anticoagulation, he returned to his work as a professional firefighter and has suffered no recurrent neurologic event.)

When attending the young adult who has had a transient ischemic attack or ischemic stroke, the clinician must consider cryptogenic stroke related to a PFO or to a hypercoagulable state in association with APS or Factor V Leiden mutation.

Cryptogenic stroke is the term applied to those patients, usually under the age of 50 years, who have suffered an acute ischemic cerebral event without an identifiable embolic source and without an identifiable large arterial atherosclerotic source. Recent clinical investigation has demonstrated that many of these ischemic events originate in an embolus that arises in a *systemic vein* in the leg or pelvis that travels to the right atrium, across a PFO into the left atrium, and ultimately, from the left ventricle to the brain.

A PFO is a flaplike valve between the right and left atria. It plays an important role in fetal development because oxygenated blood from the umbilical vein enters the right atrium. Fetal lungs are not inflated, causing a high pulmonary vascular resistance. As a result, oxygenated blood in the right atrium moves through the PFO into the left atrium and then, ultimately, into the systemic arterial circulation. After birth, hemodynamic changes in the atria close the flap and, normally, adhesions form at the site. However, in 25% of individuals the foramen ovale remains patent. PFO is common.

Because there is normally an equal blood pressure in the two atria, what might cause a venous clot moving from a leg vein into the right atrium not to move into the right ventricle, but rather, to traverse a PFO and enter the systemic circulation?

A Valsalva maneuver appears to be the most frequent explanation. During the Valsalva strain period, right atrial pressure is transiently greater than left atrial pressure. The clot in the right atrium then moves from right to left into the left atrium. In the course of daily activity, a person frequently performs a

Valsalva maneuver as he or she strains to defecate, lifts or pushes a heavy object, or has a vigorous, repetitive coughing episode. Consequently, it is thought that the ischemic cerebral event occurs when the patient, inadvertently, performs a Valsalva strain maneuver that enables a clot that happens to be in the right atrium to move through the PFO into the systemic circulation.

PFO may play an important role in the genesis of migraine headaches. Although the number of patients is small, there is suggestive data that PFO closure in migraineurs who have associated aura will significantly reduce the frequency, or even end, migrainous attacks.

Diagnosis of PFO is confirmed via transesophageal echocardiography. Agitated saline is injected into the femoral vein and the patient performs a Valsalva strain maneuver. The echocardiogram documents right to left shunting at the atrial level.

Consider the following interesting questions:

- A PFO is noted in 25% of the adult population; yet, cryptogenic stroke is very uncommon. Why?

No one knows the answer.

- The source of the paradoxical embolus is thought to be a venous clot forming in the leg. In a patient suspected of having an ischemic cerebral event caused by paradoxical embolism, how often does imaging reveal a clot in a leg vein?

The answer is that seldom is the source of embolism found in a leg or pelvic vein. Nonetheless, imaging of the veins is thought to be appropriate in the patient.

- In a patient who has a venous clot that moves to the right atrium and *no PFO* in the atrial septum, what happens to the clot?

The clot moves to the right ventricle and finally into the lung. The endothelium of the lung has an active fibrinolytic system that dissolves the clot without clinical illness. Only if the venous clot is large, or multiple, will the patient have symptoms and signs of pulmonary embolism.

Other less common causes of an ischemic brain event in a young person include hypercoagulable states associated with APS or Factor V Leiden mutation. In APS there are antibodies to plasma proteins bound to phospholipids. These antibodies are also referred to as lupus anticoagulant and anticardiolipin antibodies. APS may be primary, of unknown cause, or secondary, related to systemic lupus erythematosus. Medicines that are associated with antiphospholipid antibody production include hydralazine, quinine, amoxicillin, thiazides, propranolol, phenytoin, procainamide, oral contraceptives, and phenothiazines. (These medications are associated with the drug-induced lupus syndrome.)

The clinical presentation of APS includes venous thrombosis, arterial thrombosis, recurrent fetal loss, and thrombocytopenia. APS is associated with thrombosis in deep veins of the legs, and axillary, subclavian, and retinal veins. Approximately 10% of patients who have deep vein thrombosis (DVT) have these antibodies. Pulmonary embolism is a frequent complication. APS should be suspected in any young person who has an ischemic stroke but does not have the common risk factors. In the woman who has recurrent fetal loss (spontaneous abortion) after 10 weeks gestation, APS is an important underlying cause. Livedo reticularis, a netlike pattern of macular violaceous erythema involving legs, feet, and abdomen, is noted in 20% of APS patients. It must be recognized that livedo reticularis may be entirely benign, occurring in young women aged 20 to 40 years. In these patients, the erythema is most pronounced during cool temperature exposure and disappears with warming.

Factor V Leiden is a common mutation and is considered to be the most common cause of inherited thrombophilia, increasing the tendency to venous thromboembolism. Less commonly, prothrombin gene mutation and a deficiency in proteins C and S and antithrombin cause venous thrombosis. The major clinical manifestation of Factor V Leiden mutation is DVT and pulmonary embolism. It appears that the mutation has the greatest associated risk of venous thrombosis in those who have additive factors, including oral contraceptive intake, or who have had recent surgery, are immobilized, are pregnant, or who smoke. In children, more frequently than in young adults, this mutation may cause stroke as a result of cerebral artery thrombosis. It also is associated with recurrent fetal wastage. The screening test for Factor V Leiden mutation is the activated partial thromboplastin time.

In addition to the *inherited thrombophilias causing venous thrombosis*, note that there are two important *acquired* disorders that promote venous clotting. These include nephrotic syndrome, in which deep vein and renal vein thrombosis are relatively common, and malignancy. Oftentimes, the DVT and pulmonary embolism associated with malignancy precede the diagnosis of the neoplastic disorder. The most common malignancies associated with venous thrombosis are carcinoma of the lung, colon and rectum, pancreas, kidney, and prostate.

You must remember:
1. In the young patient who has an ischemic stroke (and is in normal sinus rhythm), consider PFO, APS, and Factor V Leiden mutation.
2. In the older patient who has DVT, consider occult malignancy as the underlying cause.

Brevity 5: Consider a Metabolic Disorder in Any Patient Who Presents with Psychiatric Disturbances. In Many Cases, the Emotional Manifestations Are Very Early Signs of the Underlying Metabolic Abnormality

Clinical vignette, Patient A: A 22-year-old woman has a 1-month history of anorexia and depression. Diligent interviewing of the patient reveals that she also has mild constipation and recurrent, vague abdominal discomfort. Laboratory evaluation shows a serum calcium concentration of 12 mg/dL. The patient is diagnosed with hyperparathyroidism, and a solitary parathyroid nodule is excised. Two months after surgery the emotional symptoms are no longer present.

The symptoms of hypercalcemia are most commonly nonspecific and include weakness, fatigue, anorexia, and depression. These emotional disturbances frequently precede the classic complications of hypercalcemia, such as nephrolithiasis and peptic ulcer. It is important to note that the emotional disturbances associated with hypercalcemia may be present while the serum calcium concentration is only mildly elevated.

Clinical vignette, Patient B: A 55-year-old woman has a 2-month history of impaired memory and depression, general apathy, loss of interest in her grandchildren, loss of libido, and 3-pound weight loss. Serum sodium concentration is 129 mEq/L and serum potassium is 5.3 mEq/L. Endocrine evaluation results in a diagnosis of chronic adrenal insufficiency (Addison's disease). Appropriate replacement with glucocorticoid and mineralocorticoid replacement was associated with resolution of the symptoms.

Psychological symptoms are ubiquitous in chronic adrenal insufficiency as in this patient. The emotional complaints occur early in Addison's disease and often predate the classic symptoms of nausea, weakness, postural lightheadedness, and the appearance of hyperpigmentation.

Clinical vignette, Patient C: A 24-year-old woman has a 3-week history of anxiety, irritability, and 3-pound weight loss, without associated tremulousness or heat intolerance. She is now 9 weeks postpartum. Laboratory studies show a serum TSH concentration of 0.03 mcU/mL and total thyroxine (T4) level of 12 mcg/dL. A diagnosis of postpartum thyroiditis (PPT) was confirmed.

PPT is considered to be a variant expression of chronic autoimmune (Hashimoto's) thyroiditis. PPT typically starts 1 to 4 months after delivery and is associated with a hyperthyroid state that lasts 2 to 8 weeks. At this time, serum thyrotropin concentration is low and serum thyroxin (T4) concentration is elevated. The disorder then progresses to a hypothyroid state that lasts 2 weeks to several months. Ultimately, the patient returns to a euthyroid status.

Subacute thyroiditis (de Quervain's) is of suspected viral etiology. Most common in young women, it is associated with painful enlargement of the thyroid gland. A hyperthyroid state occurs in half of the patients, lasts several weeks, and finally, a euthyroid status is regained. A hyperthyroid state is found in Graves' disease, toxic solitary thyroid nodule, toxic multinodular goiter, and exogenous intake of excessive thyroid hormone.

The important clinical point is that psychiatric complaints are extremely common in all disorders associated with hyperthyroidism. Anxiety, emotional lability, and worsening memory are common early symptoms for which the patient may delay seeking medical attention. Further, these symptoms often result in delayed diagnosis of the increased thyroid metabolic state.

Other metabolic disorders are associated with psychiatric disturbances. Included are chronic hypocalcemia, hypercortisolism (Cushing's disease and Cushing's syndrome), Wilson's disease, pheochromocytoma, hypothyroidism, and intermittent porphyria.

Hypercortisolism is very commonly associated with obesity, hypertension, and hyperglycemia. Of course, there are many patients who have obesity, hypertension, and hyperglycemia, but do not have hypercortisolism with its excess glucocorticoid state.

Psychiatric disturbance occurs in more than half the patients with Cushing's disease or syndrome. Common complaints include anxiety, depression, emotional lability, and panic attacks. Depression occurs in two-thirds of patients. Unlike most patients with depression who have decreased appetite, depressed patients with hypercortisolism have *increased appetite* and weight gain. An important clinical point is that the psychiatric symptom is frequently the presenting complaint to the clinician.

Chronic hypocalcemia is associated with decreased production or action of vitamin D (as in malabsorption syndrome), hypoparathyroidism, or hypomagnesemia (as occurs in chronic alcohol abuse, malabsorption syndrome, or with cisplatin therapy). Hypocalcemic patients may exhibit anxiety or depression before the neurologic manifestations of circumoral paresthesias, tetany, or positive Chvostek sign are evident. Hypoalbuminemia, as is noted in chronic, severe liver disease or in nephrotic syndrome, is associated with a decrease in total serum calcium concentration but not in ionized calcium concentration. Therefore, hypoalbuminemic patients do not have symptoms or signs of hypocalcemia.

Hypothyroid patients often have poor mental concentration, depressed mood, apathy, or social withdrawal. However, it appears that these psychiatric expressions occur when the patient has other clear manifestations of the decreased thyroid state, such as cold intolerance, pallid complexion, and dry skin. However, patients with *subclinical hypothyroidism*, defined as normal serum free thyroxine (T4) concentration with a slightly elevated serum thyrotropin (TSH) concentration, appear to have increased frequency of neurotic depression or anxiety when other clinical features of hypothyroidism are not evident.

The classic presentation of pheochromocytoma is episodic hypertension in association with profuse sweating, palpitations, and headache. Anxiety often occurs during the paroxysmal release of catecholamines from the sympathetic ganglia or adrenal medulla. During the acute anxiety, the patient will have tachycardia and hypertension.

Wilson's disease is an autosomal recessive heritable disease of cellular copper transfer. The incidence is approximately 1 case in 30,000 live births. Pathologically, copper is deposited in the liver, kidney, and brain. The clinical manifestations almost always start between the ages of 6 and 30 years. Liver involvement ranges from asymptomatic hepatic dysfunction to acute liver failure to cirrhosis with portal hypertension. Young patients whose diagnosis is not made because of liver dysfunction often present with psychiatric disturbances ranging from personality change to worsening academic performance to extrapyramidal signs, such as rigidity and bradykinesia. Serum ceruloplasmin concentration is low in most patients with Wilson's disease.

Acute intermittent porphyria (AIP) is an autosomal dominant heritable disorder in which an enzyme deficiency results in impaired heme synthesis. It is more common in women; symptoms appear to be exacerbated during the premenstrual period. Approximately 90% of persons with the inherited enzyme deficiency are clinically normal throughout life. The clinical presentation of the inherited disorder starts after puberty and is neurologic, with involvement of the peripheral, autonomic, and central nervous system. The neurologic pathophysiology causes acute abdominal pain, either generalized or local, which is the most common symptom in AIP. The pain may be severe and may be associated with nausea, vomiting, diarrhea, and ileus. Peripheral neuropathy may present with proximal muscle weakness, cranial or motor neuropathy, bulbar paralysis, or sensory neuropathy. Central nervous system neuropathology may cause seizure in acute attacks of AIP.

Many medications may precipitate acute attacks of AIP. These include angiotensin converting enzyme inhibitors, barbiturates, calcium channel blockers, ergot preparations, ketoconazole, sulfonamides, and sulfonyureas.

Here is the key clinical point germane to this topic: Psychiatric disturbances may be prominent in AIP and may be the sole expression of the inherited disease. Anxiety, hysteria, depression, agitation, delirium, and psychosis may be evident. It is estimated that as many as 1 in 500 psychiatric inpatients has AIP.

You must remember:
1. Psychiatric complaints are very common reasons for patient visits.
2. Before prescribing a psychotropic medication, the clinician must studiously consider the presence of an underlying metabolic disorder as the cause of the patient's distress.
3. Many medications may precipitate the symptoms in AIP.

Brevity 6: Always Seek a Common Denominator in Medicine

The Common Denominator in Syncope Is Cerebral Ischemia

Clinical vignette, Patient A: During venipuncture in a medical clinic, a burly 31-year-old man has sweating, nausea, and then faints. Heart rate during syncope is 44/min. The patient spontaneously awakens within 1 minute.

Clinical vignette, Patient B: A 77-year-old man with known coronary heart disease and stable angina pectoris faints during a heated, vociferous argument in a condominium association meeting. He spontaneously regains consciousness in 30 seconds.

Clinical vignette, Patient C: While running on the soccer field, an 18-year-old man suddenly collapses and faints. He quickly regains consciousness and is transported to the emergency department of the closest hospital.

Three patients; three patients who have syncopal episodes; yet, three patients with totally different medical conditions. Is there a common denominator?

Indeed, the common denominator in syncope is transient, generalized cerebral ischemia. The decreased cerebral perfusion may be caused by several different pathophysiologic mechanisms. Cardiovascular etiologies of syncope include the following:

- Arrhythmia
- Obstruction to blood flow
- Reflex mechanisms
- Orthostatic hypotension

Let us consider each of these mechanisms.

A. Syncope Resulting from Arrhythmia

Bradycardia

1. In sick sinus syndrome (brady-tachy syndrome) including sinus arrest or sinus pauses
2. Second- or third-degree atrioventricular (AV) block resulting from disease of the cardiac conduction system
3. Adverse effects of medicine, for example, calcium channel blockers, beta adrenergic blockers, digoxin

Tachycardia

1. Ventricular tachycardia
2. AF in preexcitation syndrome

   Acute myocardial ischemia is a common cause of ventricular tachycardia that results in decreased cerebral blood flow and syncope. The pathophysiologic mechanism is considered to be ischemia-induced reentry circuits in the ventricle. *Fainting in the older patient during physical exertion or during a heated argument suggests myocardial ischemia-induced arrhythmia.*

A Structurally Normal Heart

There are three conditions, all associated with a *structurally normal heart*, that are associated with syncopal attacks. They are long QT interval syndrome, preexcitation syndrome, and Brugada syndrome. Long QT interval syndrome may be a heritable (genetic) disorder or acquired; related to an electrolyte abnormality, such as hypokalemia, hypocalcemia, or hypomagnesemia; or caused by the direct effect of medication on the myocardial action potential.

This syndrome places the patient at risk for the heart rhythm to suddenly catapult into ventricular tachycardia, causing syncope or, worse, sudden cardiac death. *The key clinical point is that sympathetic nervous system stimulation appears to be the trigger for development of the life-threatening tachycardia.* Fainting in a child or adolescent during physical exertion or during a heated argument suggests congenital long QT interval. Of course, acquired long QT interval may occur at any age, but again, the paroxysmal ventricular tachycardia is triggered by sympathetic nervous system stimulation.

Preexcitation syndrome is a congenital disorder in which accessory conduction fibers (Bundle of Kent) connect the atria to the ventricles, bypassing the AV node. The electrocardiographic manifestations are short PR interval, delta wave, and wide QRS complex. Conduction of action potentials through the accessory pathways bypassing the AV node predisposes the patient to AF with very fast ventricular rates, even 300/min. The patient may then have a sudden syncopal episode. However, if the AF degenerates into *ventricular* fibrillation, sudden cardiac death occurs.

Brugada syndrome is a heritable disorder (autosomal dominant) in which there is an abnormality in sodium transport in the myocardial action potential. As a result, the patient is at risk of developing ventricular tachycardia. If self-limited, the tachyarrhythmia may cause syncope; if not, sudden cardiac death results. In most cases, Brugada syndrome clinically is expressed in persons ages 20 to 65 years, though it has been reported in a child of 3 years.

A Structurally Abnormal Heart

Let us turn our attention to syncope associated with *structural heart abnormalities*. The most common and the most important condition, because of its association with sudden cardiac death, is hypertrophic cardiomyopathy (HCM). HCM is a disorder of the sarcomere in the myocardium that is clinically characterized by inappropriate left ventricular hypertrophy, hyperdynamic left ventricular contraction, increased stiffness (or reduced compliance) of the left ventricle, and, in some cases, left ventricular outflow obstruction. To the clinician, the most significant feature of hypertrophic cardiomyopathy is its *variability*: variability in genetic mutation, anatomy, clinical features, and hemodynamics.

Many genetic mutations have been identified in HCM; it appears that most mutations involve cardiac myosin or troponin. In the majority of cases, autosomal dominant inheritance can be demonstrated. Other HCM cases are sporadic. A genetic mutation found in HCM is thought to be present in 1 in 500 persons. The frequency of this mutation does not mean that HCM is a common clinical condition. Rather, it is thought that many persons with a genetic mutation of HCM live normal or near-normal lives.

Anatomically, any portion of the left ventricle may be disproportionately hypertrophic. In some patients the hypertrophy is generalized; in others, the hypertrophy may be limited to the anterior portion of the ventricular septum, or limited to the anterior and posterior septum, or limited to the septum and lateral free wall, or, predominantly, limited to the apical area. It is puzzling, but the degree of hypertrophy does not appear related to the severity of the patient's symptoms.

The full anatomic expression of HCM may not be evident until the end of adolescent growth. Let me explain the clinical importance of this statement. For example, an 18-year-old has just been diagnosed with HCM. His siblings should undergo evaluation, including history and physical exam, electrocardiography, and echocardiography. If a 13-year-old sibling has a normal echocardiogram, the diagnosis of HCM cannot be dismissed. That sibling should have an *annual echocardiogram performed through age 18 years* and at 5-year intervals as an adult. Rarely, HCM may present clinically after age 60 years. Approximately 90% of patients diagnosed with HCM are asymptomatic and are diagnosed through family screening of diagnosed HCM patients.

The classic pathophysiologic abnormality in HCM is increased stiffness (decreased compliance) of the left ventricle. The resultant increase in left ventricular end-diastolic pressure causes elevation of the mean left atrial pressure. In turn, the elevated left atrial pressure is transmitted back to the lungs, causing interstial fluid accumulation and increased lung stiffness. The patient, then, has dyspnea. Further, some HCM patients have left ventricular outflow obstruction resulting from a combination of anatomic septal hypertrophy in conjunction with abnormal mitral leaflet motion, namely, systolic anterior motion of a mitral leaflet. This anatomic and functional disturbance impairs ejection of left ventricular blood into the aorta. This patient will have a bisferiens, or a double, carotid arterial pulse.

The three cardinal symptoms in HCM are as follows:

- Dyspnea related to the stiff left ventricle
- Angina pectoris caused by increased oxygen demand of the hypertrophic myocardium
- Syncope

Syncope in HCM may be related to three different mechanisms, all resulting in generalized cerebral ischemia. First, left ventricular outflow obstruction, as described earlier, may decrease cardiac output and cerebral blood flow. Second, the hypertrophic myocardium may become ischemic with a resultant induced ventricular tachycardia causing syncope (or sudden cardiac death). Finally, some HCM patients have inappropriate peripheral vasodilation during exertion. In these patients, exercise is not associated with the expected, normal increase in blood pressure. Rather, there is a drop in blood pressure thought to be caused by inappropriate vasodilation in nonexercising muscles. The drop in blood pressure causes cerebral ischemia and syncope.

HCM is the most common cause of sudden cardiac death in high school and college athletes. Sudden death is often the *initial clinical manifestation* of the disorder, for many of these patients did not, earlier, have any of the classic symptoms. However, in those diagnosed with HCM, identified risk factors for sudden cardiac death include family history of HCM-related sudden death, syncope not related to any other specific cause, massive (> 30 mm) ventricular hypertrophy, asymptomatic ventricular tachycardia, and abnormal blood pressure response to exercise.

Syncope and sudden cardiac death in HCM are not necessarily correlated with physical exertion. Syncope may occur with or without vigorous physical exertion. Further, only about 20% of HCM patients who die suddenly were engaged in moderate to vigorous physical activity at the time of death.

Typically, syncope due to arrhythmia is not associated with prodromal symptoms prior to the sudden loss of consciousness. (An exception is the bradycardia associated with vasovagal fainting, which is described later in the section titled "Syncope Due to Reflex Mechanisms").

Brady-tachy syndrome (sick sinus syndrome) may be intrinsic or extrinsic, the latter related to medication intake or coexisting noncardiac disease. The syndrome is characterized by alternating periods of tachycardia (usually AF or atrial flutter) and bradycardia (typically related to marked sinus bradycardia or sinus arrest). The tachyarrhythmia presents with heart failure (HF), palpitations, or angina pectoris; the bradyarrhythmic episodes are associated with syncope, near-syncope, and weakness.

Pathologically, *intrinsic* brady-tachy syndrome is associated with degeneration and fibrosis of the sinoatrial node and adjacent atrial tissue. *Extrinsic* causes include intake of medications (beta adrenergic blockers, the calcium channel blockers verapamil and diltiazem, and lithium), hypothyroidism, sleep apnea, and increased intracranial pressure.

AV block is a common cause of syncopal episodes. Second-degree AV block is characterized by intermittent failure of sinoatrial impulses to depolarize the ventricle and excite ventricular contraction. It is classified as Mobitz type I (Wenckebach) in which the conduction block occurs at the level of the AV node, or Mobitz type II in which the block is infranodal. In Mobitz I block, progressive lengthening of the PR interval occurs until a sinus beat is not conducted to the ventricle. The electrocardiographic appearance of Mobitz II block is a fixed PR interval (usually > 0.20 sec) with intermittent failure of the atrial impulse to reach the ventricle. Mobitz I AV block is temporary and reversible when related to acute inferior wall myocardial infarction (the artery to the AV node is derived from the right coronary artery), heightened vagal tone, and medications (beta adrenergic blockers, the calcium channel blockers vera-pamil and diltiazem, lithium, and digoxin). Infrequently, infectious diseases such as endocarditis and Lyme disease may produce Mobitz I AV block. Mobitz II block is not reversible and is not related to medication intake. These patients generally have a poor prognosis because of associated extensive myocardial damage.

Complete AV block (third degree) may be a result of the previously men-tioned medications and, even transiently, of increased vagal tone. Degenera-tive disease of the conduction system (Lev disease) is a common underlying etiology of complete AV block. Infiltrative disease of the myocardium, partic-ularly, amyloidosis and sarcoidosis, is a much less common cause of third degree block. Rarely, endocarditis and Lyme disease may be the underlying cause.

In second- and third-degree AV block, the inability of some or all atrial impulses to reach the ventricles causes bradycardia, decreased cardiac output, generalized cerebral ischemia, and resultant syncope.

B. Syncope Due to Obstruction to Blood Flow

- Aortic valve stenosis
- Hypertrophic cardiomyopathy
- Pulmonary embolism
- Left atrial myxoma

The classic triad of symptoms in severe aortic stenosis includes dyspnea (resulting from diastolic HF), angina pectoris (even in the absence of coro-nary artery stenosis), and syncope.

The syncope is typically *associated with exertion*. With the fixed outflow obstruction at the aortic valve, the cardiac output cannot increase as would be expected during effort. At the same time, exercise induces peripheral vasodilation that lowers blood pressure. Vasodilation in the presence of fixed cardiac output causes the syncopal episode.

Signs and symptoms of DVT in the legs may be obvious, subtle, or absent. Examination of the patient whose DVT is complicated by pul-monary embolism may reveal erythema or edema of the leg and a palpable venous cord. The most common symptoms of the pulmonary embolism are acute, pleuritic chest pain and dyspnea. Not infrequently, apprehension, hemoptysis, sweating, and cough are associated symptoms. However, if the embolus (or multiple emboli) is large enough to obstruct pulmonary blood flow, then a sudden decrease in left ventricular stroke volume results and syncope occurs.

A myxoma is an atrial tumor often attached by a stalk to the left side of the atrial septum. The myxoma may move into the mitral orifice during ventricular diastole, thereby obstructing blood flow from left atrium to ventricle. A sudden drop in stroke volume results, thus provoking syncope. At other times, the tumor may fragment, leading to systemic embolism. Echocardiography provides clear imaging of these intracardiac masses.

C. Syncope Due to Reflex Mechanisms

- Parasympathetic (neurocardiogenic or vasovagal)

Vasovagal syncope includes the common faint in which the patient, often in a disquieted state, such as during venipuncture, while experiencing body pain, or with prolonged, motionless standing, has a prodrome of nausea, sweating, and warmth immediately followed by loss of consciousness.

Heightened vagal tone plays a key role in the syncope, for hypotension and bradycardia are typically present. (Vasodepressor syncope is a variant parasympathetic-mediated form of syncope in which hypotension is present, but the heart rate is normal.) Syncope associated with specific situations, for example, swallowing (deglutition), urination (micturition), and a vigorous paroxysm of coughing (posttussive), is, similarly, thought related to increased vagal tone.

An unusual variant of syncope related to heightened vagal tone is breath-holding syncope. This occurs in children 6 months to 6 years of age. The syncope is precipitated in most cases by emotional insult, fear, or mild trauma. The breath-holding has two clinical presentations, cyanotic and pallid. In the cyanotic form, crying precedes breath-holding. The child then becomes limp, blue, and faints. Generalized seizing may occur. In the pallid presentation, the child stops breathing, becomes pale and limp, faints, and may have clonic contractions and urinary incontinence. Consultation with a pediatric neurologist is generally indicated to differentiate breath-holding syncope from a primary seizure disorder.

D. Syncope Due to Orthostatic Hypotension

- Impaired sympathetic (adrenergic) reflexes
- Hypovolemia
- Adverse medicine response

The sympathetic reflex arc plays an integral role in regulation of blood pressure and cardiac output. *Normally*, assumption of the standing position from recumbency or sitting causes a prompt, initial drop in blood pressure. The initial hypotension is followed by carotid baroreceptor activation that results in efferent sympathetic stimulation. The heightened sympathetic tone produces an increase in heart rate and constriction of arterioles and veins. The blood pressure increases as a result of the arteriolar constriction increasing systemic vascular resistance. At the same time, stimulation of sympathetic fibers that innervate the heart results in an increase in heart rate and contractility. Resultantly, enhanced propulsion of blood contributes to an increased blood pressure upon standing in conjunction with increased cardiac output.

Consequently, in the normal person, assumption of the standing position is associated with a slight decrease in systolic blood pressure, a slight increase in diastolic pressure, and a modest increase in heart rate. *Mean arterial pressure is the same in the standing as in the recumbent position.*

In the patient who has adrenergic insufficiency, either primary or secondary (as is common in diabetic autonomic neuropathy), assumption of the standing position does not result in arteriolar constriction or increase in heart rate. Here is a common clinical vignette:

> **An elderly patient with type 2 diabetes mellitus has lightheadedness, dimmed vision, and feeling of impending faint upon rising from bed. Blood pressure in the sitting position is 122/76 mm Hg with pulse of 78/min. Upon standing, blood pressure is 84/60 mm Hg with pulse of 80/min.**

What is the pathophysiologic mechanism that is causing symptoms and the observed hemodynamic response in the adrenergic dysfunction? Upon standing, note that both systolic and diastolic blood pressure significantly decrease (orthostatic hypotension), but heart rate does not increase—all resulting from an impaired sympathetic response to assumption of upright posture. The deficient sympathetic reflex response does not result in the expected normal compensatory response, namely, an increased heart rate and arteriolar constriction that would maintain a normal blood pressure in the standing position. Clinically, orthostatic hypotension causing syncope due to autonomic insufficiency is very common, particularly in diabetic patients.

In contrast, orthostatic hypotension is very common in patients who are hypovolemic. The decreased circulating blood volume may be a result of excessive diuresis, hemorrhage, or endocrinopathy, such as chronic adrenal insufficiency with hypovolemia related to a deficiency in mineralocorticoid hormones. Orthostatic hypotension is related to the abnormally low circulating blood volume. In these patients, the sympathetic nervous system is intact. Therefore, with assumption of the standing position, systolic and diastolic blood pressure drops, but the *heart rate significantly increases* (12 to 20 beats per minute) because the sympathetic reflexes and baroreceptor stimulation are intact. Therefore, heart rate increases in an appropriate compensatory response to the orthostatic hypotension.

Note the important clinical difference: *In orthostatic hypotension related to adrenergic (sympathetic) dysfunction, the drop in blood pressure is not associated with an increase in heart rate. In orthostatic hypotension due to hypovolemia, the drop in blood pressure is associated with a compensatory increase in heart rate.*

An Important Clinical Point That Is Correlated with Syncope of Any Etiology: "All That Seizes Is Not Epilepsy"

> Clinical vignette: A 48-year-old woman was walking in a mall pushing a baby stroller when she suddenly collapsed and fainted. Witnesses noted jerking of the legs bilaterally during the brief period of unconsciousness. The patient quickly awakened and was transported to the emergency department. Brain imaging studies were normal. A diagnosis of epilepsy was made. Anti-epileptic medication was prescribed. Two months later the patient had acute, fulminating hepatic failure due to the anti-epileptic medication. Liver transplantation was performed.

Careful review of the medical record revealed that the electrocardiogram taken in the emergency department after the acute event showed that the patient had normal sinus rhythm, a very long PR interval (first-degree AV block), with complete right bundle branch block and left anterior hemiblock. Clearly, electrocardiography showed evidence of markedly impaired AV and intraventricular conduction, which placed the patient at high risk for complete (third-degree) heart block.

Simply put, this patient was at very high risk of having an episode of complete heart block causing syncope, not having an epileptic attack. Appropriate cardiac evaluation would have demonstrated the need for a permanent cardiac pacemaker.

Syncope of any etiology may be associated with jerking motion of the extremities. Do not catapult to a diagnosis of epilepsy without careful consideration of whether the patient may have had a syncopal episode with secondary muscle jerking.

Let us continue on the theme "All that seizes is not epilepsy."

> Clinical vignette: It occurred many years ago; I was in the very first week of my clinical practice. I happened to be seated in the physicians' lounge of the hospital having a cup of coffee. A young

man, unknown to me and in an obvious state of disquietude, sat down at the same small table. Speaking quickly, he told me his name and that he was a neurologist. "I don't understand," he cried. Clearly, I had no idea what he meant.

Without my inquiry, he volunteered that the previous day he had taken his oral examination for certification as a specialist in neurology. He had failed the examination and was distraught. Again, there was no time for me to utter a word. "Here's the case. Where did I go wrong?"

The specialty board examiner presented him with a case: A 14-year-old boy is transported to the emergency department and is having generalized seizures. The examiner asked, "How would you treat the patient?" The young neurologist, the test candidate now seated opposite me, responded that he would administer intravenous phenytoin. The examiner said that the seizures continue. "Now what would you do?" An increased dose of phenytoin; yet the seizures continue. Intravenous administration of phenobarbital; yet the seizures continue. "Now what would you do?" "I would take the patient to the operating room and have the anesthesiologist administer general anesthesia" (remember, this was 5 decades ago).

The examiner stood up, and without saying a word, slapped his hand on the table and hurriedly walked out of the room. A moment later, he returned, said, "You failed," and left.

"Where did I go wrong?" the neurologist plaintively repeated the question. Softly, I whispered, "Hypoglycemia." He threw his head back, closed his eyes, and cried.

"All that seizes is not epilepsy."

The Common Denominator in Cor Pulmonale Is Pulmonary Hypertension Due to Increased Pulmonary Vascular Resistance

Cor pulmonale is heart disease secondary to lung disease. The lung disease may be vascular, for example, multiple pulmonary emboli; parenchymal, for example, chronic bronchitis or interstitial pulmonary fibrosis; or pneumonioconiosis, for example, asbestosis or chronic beryllium disease. In each of these conditions, there is destruction of the pulmonary vascular bed. Massive obesity and hypoventilation (Pickwickian syndrome) are associated with alveolar hypoxia that causes pulmonary vasoconstriction.

Whether the mechanism is vasoconstriction or the physical obliteration of the pulmonary vascular bed, the common denominator is an increase in pulmonary vascular resistance that produces an increase in pulmonary artery pressure (pulmonary hypertension) and, ultimately, right heart failure (right HF).

Right heart failure due to pulmonary hypertension from lung disease is cor pulmonale. Signs of right HF include left parasternal lift, elevated jugular venous pressure, congestive hepatomegaly (smooth, tender, enlarged liver), modest ascites, and peripheral edema.

The most common cause of right HF is chronic systolic left heart failure. This is not, however, cor pulmonale because the right HF is not due to lung disease. Finally, note that in the typical patient who has emphysema (in contrast to chronic bronchitis), pulmonary artery pressure is normal or near normal. As a result, emphysema patients do not develop cor pulmonale.

A Dilated Left Atrium Is a Common Denominator in Atrial Fibrillation

AF is the most common sustained, significant, and problematic arrhythmia in clinical practice. AF is associated with reduced quality of life, serious morbidity, and increased mortality. Left atrial dilatation (increased left atrial dimension) is commonly seen in patients with AF.

A dilated left atrium leads to AF. Oppositely, AF leads to a dilated left atrium. A dilated left atrium is common in patients who have mitral valve disease (stenosis or regurgitation), mitral annulus calcification, hypertensive heart disease, and atherosclerotic heart disease, especially in those who have sustained a myocardial infarction. In each of these conditions, there is stretching of the left atrial walls that causes left atrial dilatation that, in turn, appears to be a key factor in the genesis of AF.

There is evidence that AF itself results in left atrial dilatation. This may explain why *paroxysmal* AF commonly progresses to *chronic* AF. Further, this may explain why electrical or chemical cardioversion of AF is more difficult in patients with a longer duration of AF.

Ischemia of Muscle Is the Common Denominator in the "Claudications"

The term *claudication* is linguistically derived from the Latin word meaning "cramping." *Angina* is also derived from the Latin, meaning "strangling." Whether it be anginal discomfort in the chest or cramping in the leg, ischemia of muscle is the unifying pathophysiologic mechanism.

The key clinical point is that there are many claudications. The common denominator of muscle ischemia and claudication relate to the following structures:

- Heart

- Leg
- Arm
- Jaw
- Intestine
- Uterus

Cardiac claudication, of course, is angina pectoris. The myocardial ischemia may result from myocardial oxygen demand outstripping oxygen supply, as is typical in the patient who has atherosclerotic heart disease or left ventricular hypertrophy of any etiology. In these conditions, myocardial ischemia causes ST segment depression in the electrocardiogram.

Conversely, myocardial ischemia and angina pectoris may occur when oxygen supply is reduced at a time when myocardial demand is normal. This is typical of variant angina (Prinzmetal angina) in which coronary artery spasm is the underlying mechanism producing cardiac ischemia. Remember, during anginal discomfort in variant angina the ST segments are elevated.

Claudication involving the lower extremity may be due to aortoiliac occlusive arterial disease. These patients have hip and buttocks aching with walking (Leriche's syndrome). Almost always, in the male the vascular disease causes impotence. Further, atherosclerotic stenosis or occlusion of the common femoral artery causes claudication of the thigh. Superficial femoral artery stenosis typically causes cramping in the upper two-thirds of the calf; exertional cramping of the lower third of the calf is usually due to popliteal artery aneurysm or stenosis.

Claudication involving the arm occurs in one-third of patients who have subclavian steal syndrome. This disorder is due to atherosclerotic subclavian artery stenosis proximal to the origin of the vertebral artery. In these patients, there is always a significant difference in systolic blood pressure between the normal and affected arm. In my experience, the systolic blood pressure in the affected arm (the side of the arterial stenosis) is always at least 20 mm Hg lower than in the normal arm.

Patients with subclavian steal syndrome generally have *either* neurologic symptoms or arm symptoms. Neurologic symptoms that may be resulting from retrograde flow in the affected vertebral artery ("steal") include the classic symptoms of vertebrobasilar artery insufficiency:

- Dizziness or vertigo
- Ataxia
- Blurring of vision in both eyes or diplopia
- Tinnitus

Exercise involving the arm on the affected side may cause arm cramping (claudication) in addition to coolness and paresthesias or, occasionally, numbness.

A special type of subclavian steal syndrome may be termed "internal mammary-coronary steal." Note that in the following case, the development of subclavian artery stenosis presents as recurrent angina pectoris, not with arm claudication or vertebrobasilar artery insufficiency symptoms.

> **Clinical vignette: A patient has undergone left internal mammary artery bypass grafting for treatment of angina pectoris. Two years later, the angina pectoris recurs. The clinical impression is that the patient has developed a new coronary atherosclerotic stenosis.**
>
> **Examination shows blood pressure in the right arm is 130/82 mm Hg; in the left arm, 104/82 mm Hg. What is going on in this case? The patient has developed new left subclavian artery stenosis (ipsilateral side to the graft) that is causing reappearance of angina pectoris. The new left subclavian artery stenosis is causing retrograde blood flow in the grafted internal mammary artery (steal).**

A key clinical point that you must remember: It is imperative to take the blood pressure in both arms of all patients, particularly those with known atherosclerotic disease. If you do not take bilateral blood pressure measurements in the patient with prior internal mammary artery graft, recrudescence of angina pectoris will be attributed to the development of a new coronary artery atheromatous stenosis rather than the correct cause, namely, development of subclavian artery stenosis.

Claudication of the jaw is a common symptom in the patient who has giant cell arteritis, occurring in 50% of cases. Often, jaw claudication is an early symptom. It may be unilateral or bilateral. The aching discomfort is felt while chewing and is relieved in minutes by rest. This discomfort is mimicked by the discomfort noted by the patient who has temporomandibular joint pain. However, claudication is clearly differentiated from jaw fatigability without discomfort that is characteristic of myasthenia gravis.

Other symptoms of giant cell arteritis include headache, fever, visual loss, fatigue, and weight loss. Please refer to the section titled "Stroke *and* Fever" in Chapter 2, "The Most Important Word in Diagnosis: *And.*"

Intestinal claudication or chronic mesenteric ischemia of the small bowel is usually due to atherosclerotic stenosis in the superior mesenteric or celiac artery. Patients have crampy, dull postprandial pain in the epigastrium and upper abdomen that starts within the first hour after eating and subsides within 2 hours. Patients who have intestinal claudication typically have recognized atherosclerotic heart or cerebrovascular disease.

There is one more claudication, one that is termed "neurogenic claudication" or more properly, "pseudoclaudication." It is not related to ischemia; rather, it is due to osteophytic narrowing of the lumbar spinal canal. Pseudoclaudication may produce buttock or leg discomfort with walking; most commonly, it involves the calf or distal lower extremity. It resolves with rest similar to vascular claudication. In contrast to ischemia-induced leg discomfort, at times, neurogenic claudication will cause discomfort while the patient is standing still.

To differentiate vascular from neurogenic claudication, consider the following:

- Pulses are absent in vascular but are often normal in neurogenic.
- Pain with cough or sneezing occurs only in neurogenic.
- Neurogenic patients often have a dermatomal sensory deficit.
- In 30% of cases, neurogenic patients have limited straight leg raising.

Is There a Common Denominator in Clubbing? It Seems More and More Likely That There Is One

Clubbing is noted in patients who have disparate diseases that include cyanotic congenital heart disease, chronic inflammatory disorders, and malignant neoplasia. Specific diseases in which clubbing occurs include these:

- Tetralogy of Fallot
- Transposition of the great arteries
- Infective endocarditis
- Cystic fibrosis, empyema, tuberculosis, lung abscess, and bronchiectasis
- Primary and metastatic lung cancer
- Inflammatory bowel disease
- Cirrhosis
- Celiac disease

Clubbing is not associated with chronic obstructive lung disease or sarcoidosis, even when the sarcoidosis is associated with pulmonary fibrosis. *Never ascribe clubbing to chronic obstructive lung disease.*

Vascular endothelial growth factor (VEGF) is the single biologic agent that may be the common denominator that links these disorders to clubbing of fingers and toes. VEGF stimulates vascular growth in tissues as is found in clubbed digits.

VEGF is increased in conditions that are all associated with clubbing:

- Tissue hypoxia of any etiology

- Chronic inflammation
- Malignancy

In disorders in which hypoxia or inflammation is present, normal tissues produce VEGF. However, in malignancy the tumor cells produce the VEGF.

It is fascinating how such unrelated medical disorders have the same sign, clubbing, and how VEGF appears to be the common denominator linking them.

Alpha Fetoprotein: A Common Denominator in Tumor Markers

Worldwide, it is estimated that 12% of all deaths are due to cancer. Understandably, intensive research is directed toward finding serum markers that indicate the presence of a specific neoplasm or the very high likelihood of a person developing that tumor.

CA 125 and CA 19-9, carcinoembryonic antigen (CEA), and prostate-specific antigen (PSA) are well known to the public. Alpha fetoprotein (AFP) is, perhaps, less well known, but is an important common denominator in certain tumors.

Tumor markers are proteins. Cancer is essentially the unregulated growth of normal tissue; thus, both nonmalignant and malignant tissues may produce these proteins. A number of these protein markers are, in fact, tumor antigens. These antigens include CEA, AFP, and the cancer antigens CA 125 and CA 19-9.

Markers are considered to be *cancer specific*, meaning that they are directly associated with the presence of neoplasms. Cancer-specific markers include CEA, CA 19-9, and CA 125. Other markers are considered to be *tissue specific*, meaning that they are not directly related to a neoplasm, but are associated with certain tissues that are undergoing neoplastic change. AFP and PSA are tissue-specific markers. Further, AFP is considered to be an *oncofetal* antigen, meaning that it is present in normal fetal tissue and diminishes to undetectable levels in normal humans.

What Is the Common Denominator in AFP?

- Serum levels of AFP are elevated in 95% of males who have testicular germ cell gonadal tumors.
- An increasing serum AFP concentration in a patient with cirrhosis raises concern for the development of hepatocellular carcinoma.
- An elevated maternal serum AFP raises suspicion of a neural tube defect in the fetus. An ultrasound examination and amniocentesis should then be performed to determine whether the neural tube defect

is, in fact, present. I have not found an explanation why the AFP marker is elevated in neural tube defects.

Is There a Common Denominator That Links Disparate Functions and Conditions?

Are the following functions and conditions linked in some way?

- Valvular heart stenosis
- Mood and memory
- Sleep and wakefulness
- Migraine headaches
- Appetite
- Pain perception
- Bowel contractility
- Temperature regulation

Yes, there is a common denominator. It is a hormone called serotonin, also known as 5-hydroxytryptamine (5-HT).

Important clinical questions immediately come to mind. What is serotonin and what does it do? How can one hormone have such widely different physiologic effects? How does one hormone accomplish a response in so many different tissues?

The ubiquitous expression of serotonin is related to the fact that there are *at least seven major families of serotonin receptors*. Each family of receptors has its own structure, its own pharmacology, and its own functional property. The receptors all have the basic "5-HT" label, followed by a suffix (e.g., 5-HT 1, 5-HT 2). The 5-HT 1 and 5-HT 5 receptors are in the brain; 5-HT 2 receptors are in heart and stomach; the 5-HT 4 receptors are in the bowel.

Serotonin is a hormone derived from the amino acid tryptophan that has both central and peripheral physiologic effects. Serotonin is synthesized primarily (95%) in the enterochromaffin cells of the gut mucosa and to a lesser degree in the brain and in mast cells of large bronchi. The hormone synthesized in the gut mucosa is released into the circulation where it is stored in platelets.

Serotonin is a neurotransmitter (along with acetylcholine, norepinephrine, dopamine, gamma amino butyric acid, glutamate, and glycine) secreted into the parenchyma of the brain. The hormone's effect in different areas of the brain is expressed in many psychologic functions, for example, inhibiting aggressive behavior and anxiety, promoting sleep, and elevating mood. Serotonin receptors in the brain stem and in the dorsal nerve roots modulate pain perception; activation of these receptors lessens the patient's awareness of painful stimuli.

Serotonin plays an important role in migraine headaches. It appears that the final event leading to migraine pain is release of inflammatory vasodilators at the peripheral nerve endings of the trigeminal nerve (cranial nerve V) on vessels of the meninges and scalp. Release of serotonin from platelets is thought to promote this pathway. Platelet concentration of serotonin is increased before a migraine headache; during the migraine headache the serotonin concentration in the platelets is low. The action of the SSRIs (or triptans) in treatment of acute migraine is still somewhat ill defined. One beneficial action of the triptans is to stimulate 5-HT 1 receptors that reduce dural arterial vasodilation and inflammation. Additionally, the triptans stimulate the 5-HT 1 serotonin receptors in the brain stem, which reduces the awareness of pain.

Plasma concentrations of the serotonin precursor, tryptophan, are lower in patients who suffer from major depression compared to healthy, normal subjects. The beneficial pharmacologic effect of the SSRIs in treatment of depression is to potentiate serotonin's effect on brain receptors. It is clearly recognized that there is an increased prevalence of depression in children and adolescents who have type 1 diabetes mellitus. The explanation may be significantly related to the fact that plasma serotonin levels are lower in these patients compared to nondiabetic subjects.

Medications that block secretions of serotonin cause depression. In contrast, medications that increase serotonin activity in the brain lessen depression. This explains the effectiveness of SSRI medication in treatment of depression. It is clinically estimated that three-quarters of patients with depression are effectively treated with SSRIs that block the uptake of serotonin at nerve endings.

Serotonin increases bowel contractility and secretions; an elevated level of serotonin, as in carcinoid syndrome, causes the diarrhea characteristic of that tumor. In the heart, serotonin is released from platelets in response to a damaged endothelium as occurs in atheromatous plaque rupture. Serotonin's release from platelets increases the synthesis of thromboxane A2, whose local vascular effect is platelet aggregation and vasoconstriction, thus promoting acute thrombosis.

What Is the Link Between Serotonin and Valvular Heart Disease?

Patients who have carcinoid syndrome have a classic triad of symptoms: flushing, diarrhea, and wheezing. The flushing and wheezing are related to the tumor's release of histamine, not serotonin. It is the serotonin that causes the secretory diarrhea. Interestingly, carcinoid tumors that arise in the intestine do not cause *carcinoid syndrome* unless liver metastases are present. However, patients who have bronchial carcinoids may manifest the syndrome without metastases.

Further, it is known that patients with carcinoid syndrome often have valvular heart disease, most notably pulmonic and tricuspid stenosis. The *same fibrotic valvular disease* is noted in the following patients:

- Patients who ingest ergot alkaloid medication, such as ergotamine, methysergide, pergolide, and cabergoline (note the *ergo* in medication nomenclature)
- Patients who ingest the anorectic medicine combination fenfluramine and phentermine ("fen-phen")

Here are the key clinical points that you must know:

- The specific family of serotonin receptor called 5-HT 2 stimulates fibroblast growth and deposition of fibrous tissue on the valvular endocardium.
- The ergot medicines, the anorectic medications fenfluramine and phentermine, and carcinoid syndrome all share a single feature—they all increase serotonin levels and all stimulate the 5-HT 2 receptor. Therefore, they all cause valvular stenosis that predominantly affects the tricuspid and pulmonic valves.
- SSRIs that increase serotonin activity in the brain *do not stimulate 5-HT 2 receptors* and, therefore, do not cause valvular stenosis.
- Triptans, important medicine used in the therapy of acute migraine headaches, are serotonin agonists that increase serotonin activity in the brain. Again, triptans *do not stimulate 5-HT 2 receptors* and, therefore, do not cause valvular stenosis.

You must remember:
1. There are clinically important common denominators in patients who have syncope, cor pulmonale, AF, clubbing, and elevated serum alpha fetoprotein.
2. Serotonin is a common denominator in patients with emotional and eating disorders, right heart valvular stenosis, and the triad of flushing, wheezing, and diarrhea.

Are There Common Denominators in Heart Failure?

HF is a cardiac dysfunction manifest by an inability to achieve a cardiac output adequate to meet the metabolic demands of the body at normal ventricular filling pressures.

Why is the definition of HF so complex, combining *cardiac output* with *ventricular filling pressures*? The answer is that the single definition of HF includes:

- Different symptoms
- Different physical signs
- Different pathophysiology
- Different therapy

There are, in fact, many types of HFs. Think, for a moment, of the clinician addressing a patient in HF. The patient may indeed exhibit varied symptoms and signs associated with the following:

- Left heart systolic HF
- Left heart diastolic HF
- Combined systolic and diastolic HF
- Right HF
- Biventricular HF
- High cardiac output HF
- HF with normal circulating blood volume
- HF with increased circulating blood volume
- HF associated with arrhythmia
- HF associated with acute myocardial infarction/acute ischemia
- An asymptomatic patient with left ventricular dysfunction

We may return to the original question: Are there common denominators in heart failure? Yes.

Common denominator 1. Cardiac chambers have the ability to alter their size and configuration to a chronic change in hemodynamic load. This is called *remodeling*. Increased preload means an increase in the volume of blood in a ventricle at end-diastole, a moment before ventricular contraction begins. Increased preload leads to ventricular dilation.

Increased afterload means increased resistance to outflow of blood from a ventricle during systole. Afterload on the left ventricle, then, relates to systemic blood pressure and presence of aortic valve stenosis. *Increased afterload leads to ventricular hypertrophy.*

Common denominator 2. All patients with HF demonstrate activation of compensatory neurohumoral systems. The purpose of the neurohumoral systems is to maintain an adequate cardiac output and perfusion pressure (arterial blood pressure). These neurohumoral systems include the following:

- Sympathetic nervous system
- Renin angiotensin aldosterone system
- Tissue renin angiotensin system

- Vasopressin (antidiuretic hormone)
- Brain natriuretic peptide
- Endothelin
- Kallikrein-kinin
- Prostaglandins
- Nitric oxide

Neurohumoral systems are initially beneficial in maintaining an adequate cardiac output and blood pressure, but ultimately, they are destructive, leading to premature mortality.

Common denominator 3. Dyspnea on a *cardiac basis* is pathophysiologically due to a noncompliant (stiff) left ventricle that causes an increase in mean left atrial pressure. The left atrial pressure is transmitted back through the pulmonary veins to the pulmonary capillaries. The lungs become congested and stiff—and the patient experiences breathlessness. This is diastolic heart failure.

All patients who have diastolic heart failure have a stiff left ventricle.

Common denominator 4. Weakness on a *cardiac basis* is pathophysiologically due to impaired vigor of left ventricular contraction. Stroke volume and cardiac output are reduced. Reduced arterial flow to muscles causes the patient to sense weakness. This is systolic heart failure.

All patients with systolic heart failure have a decreased cardiac output due to reduced vigor of left ventricular power.

Common denominator 5. In any patient who presents with HF, *look for precipitating factors*. These include the following:

- Ischemia/infarction. The first question the clinician must consider in the patient with HF is, "Is the heart failure due to ischemia or infarction?" If the answer is yes, *the clinician must treat the ischemia and the HF*.
- Medications that reduce contractility
- Calcium channel blockers
- Beta adrenergic blockers
- Doxorubicin
- Discontinuation of medication
- Sodium-retaining medications
- Acute blood pressure rise in the normotensive patient

- Superimposed infection, for example, pneumonia
- Anemia
- Acidosis of any etiology (metabolic or respiratory)
- Emotional stress
- High environmental temperature

You must remember:
1. While HF has multiple pathophysiologic mechanisms, there are still common denominators.
2. Understanding these common denominators enables the clinician to better define and treat HF.

Brevity 7: Flushing

Flushing is a ubiquitous symptom in medicine. It is related to emotion, ingestion of food or medicine, neoplasia, endocrine imbalance, and dermatologic disorders. Further, its causes are age-related.

Clinical vignette, Healthy Individual A: A 22-year-old woman appears for her medical school interview. When addressing the first question, "Why do you want to be a doctor?" her face, neck, and upper anterior chest become intensely flushed without associated sweating.

Clinical vignette, Healthy Individual B: A 51-year-old woman in early menopause awakens an average of three times a night with an intense feeling of body heat, sweating, and flushing. During the daytime, she experiences very few of these episodes.

Clinical vignette, Patient C: A 34-year-old man has the sudden onset of palpitations. In the emergency department, blood pressure is 106/68, pulse 190/min/regular, and respirations 21/min. Electrocardiography reveals paroxysmal supraventricular tachycardia. Immediately after receiving intravenous adenosine, the patient becomes flushed, but normal sinus rhythm is restored.

Clinical vignette, Patient D: A 71-year-old man has a 3-week history of recurrent flushing. During the same time, he has noted that the veins on the left side of his scrotum are dilated and prominent. He now has two episodes of gross hematuria. Urologic investigation reveals a left renal cell carcinoma that has invaded the left renal vein.

Clinical vignette, Patient E: A 62-year-old man has flushing of his face that begins approximately 10 minutes after ingestion of alcohol or spicy foods. Examination shows telangiectasia and papules on the nose and cheeks. The clinical diagnosis is rosacea.

The vignettes illustrate that the cutaneous vasodilation known to lay persons and clinicians as flushing is common and has many disparate causes. Flushing may be entirely benign as in the interview candidate or may represent a fatal disease as in the patient with renal cell carcinoma whose tumor has invaded the left renal vein. (Remember that the left gonadal vein draining the scrotum empties into the *left renal vein*, so a new left varicocele should raise suspicion of left renal cell carcinoma.)

The complexity of medical practice, its richness, and its challenge relate to the fact that so many conditions have multiple causes, some entirely benign that require only reassurance of the patient, while other causes are life-threatening and require intensive intervention. Flushing is one such example; another is syncope. As has been discussed, syncope may be entirely benign as in the common vasovagal faint, or syncope may result from life-threatening, malignant ventricular arrhythmia.

Headache, snoring, and cough all may be entirely benign or related to serious illness.

Causes of Flushing

The causes of flushing are divided into *physiologic, medicine-induced, and disease states.*

Physiologic Causes of Flushing
- Emotion
- Fever
- Menopause and pregnancy
- Ingestion of hot drinks or spicy food
- Ingestion of alcohol

Medicine Causing Flushing
- Niacin
- Adenosine
- Calcium channel blockers
- Nitroglycerin and amyl nitrite
- Levodopa
- Tamoxifen
- Sildenafil
- Hydralazine

- Vancomycin
- Cyclosporine, doxorubicin, cisplatin, interferon
- Contrast media

Disease States Causing Flushing
- Anaphylaxis
- Rosacea
- Dermatomyositis
- Seborrheic dermatitis
- Carcinoid syndrome
- Medullary carcinoma of thyroid
- Renal cell carcinoma
- Mastocytosis
- Pheochromocytoma
- Migraine, cluster headache, and trigeminal neuralgia—unilateral flushing
- Brain tumors affecting the third ventricle

With so many potential causes, how does the clinician approach the patient who has flushing?

First, quickly determine whether the symptom is of physiologic origin or is due to medication.

Second, determine whether the flushing is associated with diarrhea because this symptom is characteristic of medullary carcinoma of the thyroid, mastocytosis, and carcinoid syndrome.

Third, assess for the presence of skin lesions, which should raise suspicion of mastocytosis or dermatomyositis. Seborrhea and rosacea will be clearly evident; skin biopsy may be necessary to establish the diagnosis of mastocytosis. Patients with dermatomyositis typically have muscle weakness with an associated abnormality in serum muscle antibodies, for example, creatine kinase, aldolase, and lactic dehydrogenase, in addition to the presence of antinuclear antibodies in serum.

Episodic or persistent hypertension suggests pheochromocytoma. Microscopic hematuria suggests renal cell carcinoma with flushing related to an associated paraneoplastic syndrome.

You must remember:
1. Flushing is a common symptom.
2. You must first exclude physiologic or medicine-related causes of flushing. Your history must carefully include all over-the-counter health supplements.
3. Finally, seek the less common, organic diseases associated with flushing.

Brevity 8: Heart Rate Is Not the Most Important Element in Cardiopulmonary Fitness

> Clinical vignette: Recently, I was working out in the exercise room in the condominium in which I reside. A resident in the building came to me and said, "Isn't it true that a measure of physical fitness is getting the heart rate up high?" I nodded, but before I could fully respond, he continued, "Then, I must be healthy because I get a real fast heart rate in the sauna."

Quite simply, the role of the cardiovascular system is to maintain an adequate cardiac output and perfusion pressure. The respiratory system has two elemental goals, namely, to deliver oxygen to the tissues for cell metabolism and to remove carbon dioxide to maintain a normal chemical (i.e., pH) balance.

With physical exertion, an increase in cardiac output and in ventilation is necessary to preserve cellular oxygenation and maintain acid–base balance. The heart rate increase associated with aerobic exercise is a hemodynamic correlate of the body's oxygen uptake. However, an increase in heart rate alone is not indicative of aerobic capacity. An increase in heart rate associated with anxiety, relaxing in a heated sauna, or ingestion of a sympathomimetic or anticholinergic medicine does not impart cardiopulmonary fitness.

Most regrettably, cardiopulmonary fitness requires physical work.

There is an interesting corollary, however. Cardiovascular fitness may be reached without a significant increase in heart rate. Patients with fixed-rate cardiac pacemakers and those with blunted heart rate responses to exercise due to intake of beta adrenergic blocker medications can still achieve an exercise-induced increase in metabolic rate and state of cardiopulmonary fitness.

Brevity 9: Think of the Chronology of a Heart Murmur

The traditional and careful evaluation of a heart murmur includes the following assessments:

- Timing in the cardiac cycle
- Location
- Radiation
- Quality

- Duration
- Influence by maneuvers, such as change in body position, breathing, Valsalva strain, or squatting

Another clinically important factor in the evaluation of a murmur is what I call its "chronology." In other words, how has the murmur changed in relation to the patient's clinical status?

Clinical vignette, Patient A: A 59-year-old man has known chronic mitral regurgitation with a holosystolic murmur. Upon follow-up cardiac examination, you are now aware that the holosystolic murmur is distinctly softer than in the past and of shorter duration.

This may be an important clue signifying that systolic left ventricular function is worsening because a feebly contracting ventricle is unable to generate the same degree of turbulent flow as in the past. If, however, this patient's left ventricular function later improves with therapy, the improved hemodynamics will have an auscultatory correlation. The murmur will increase in intensity and duration.

Clinical vignette, Patient B: A 26-year-old man has acute viral myocarditis. A new murmur of mitral regurgitation is heard. What is the etiology of the murmur?

The impaired contractile strength of the myofibrils causes the left ventricle to dilate. This, in turn, causes disruption of the mitral valve apparatus, onset of mitral regurgitation, and appearance of the murmur. Clearly, the new mitral regurgitant murmur is not due to a primary defect in the valve leaflets themselves. Rather, it is the dilated left ventricle, with its secondary effect on the papillary muscles, chordae tendineae, and mitral valve ring, that is responsible for the murmur. If recovery is associated with improved left ventricular systolic function, the ventricle will reduce in chamber volume and the murmur may disappear.

Clinical vignette, Patient C: An 81-year-old woman has known calcific aortic stenosis due to degeneration of the valve cusps. You now note the murmur to be softer in intensity. What is the pathophysiologic significance of the softening of the murmur?

The murmur intensity is lessening because the hypertrophic left ventricle is now losing contractile power. Stroke volume and ejection fraction are decreasing; therefore, there is a reduction in the ability of the left ventricle to generate a turbulent flow across the aortic valve.

Clinical vignette, Patient D: A 22-year-old man has infectious endocarditis of the aortic valve. Six hours after admission, the diastolic murmur of aortic regurgitation is softer in intensity. What does this mean?

The murmur is decreasing in intensity because left ventricular function is worsening. It seems paradoxical, but the softer murmur means that the patient is sicker. The diastolic murmur is getting softer because the left ventricular end-diastolic pressure is rising. There is now a lesser gradient between aorta pressure and ventricular diastolic pressure. A reduced gradient results in less turbulent regurgitant flow and a softer murmur.

Remember this clinical point: *The intensity of a heart murmur is not simply dependent upon the anatomic severity of a valvular or congenital defect.* Rather, the murmur is dependent upon physiologic factors including ventricular function and, at times, systemic or pulmonary vascular resistance. The chronology of the murmur reflects these physiologic changes.

Brevity 10: Make It Easier to Remember

I have long believed that students expend far too much time and energy *memorizing* information. Indeed, there is so much to learn. Therefore, I always sought clues to help me remember clinically important material. I share with you a few examples of how I made remembering so much easier.

Remember That the Suffix and, at Times, the Prefix, of a Medicine's Generic Name Indicates the Class of That Medication

Here are some important suffixes:

-olol = Beta adrenergic blocker
Examples: propranolol, metoprolol, esmolol, acebutol
Note that *alol* does not indicate a pure beta blocker.
Alol, as in labetalol, is a combined beta and alpha adrenergic blocker.

-statin = HMG-CoA reductase inhibitor
Examples: simvastatin, pravastatin, atorvastatin, fluvastatin

-am = Benzodiazepams
Examples: diazepam, lorazepam, flurazepam, temazepam, midazolam, alprazolam
Exceptions: chlordiazepoxide, clorazepate

-cyclines = Tetracyclines
Examples: demeclocycline, chlortetracycline, minocycline

-cillin = Penicillins

Examples: penicillin G, cloxacillin, dicloxacillin, nafcillin, amoxicillin, ampicillin, mezlocillin, piperacillin, ticarcillin

-sartin = Angiotensin II receptor blocker

Examples: candesartan, eprosartan, olmesartan, valsartan, telmisartan, irbesartan

-pril = Angiotensin converting enzyme inhibitor

Examples: benazepril, captopril, enalapril, fosinopril, moexipril, quinapril, ramipril, trandolapril

-zide = Thiazides

Examples: hydrochlorothiazide, polythiazide, methyclothiazide, hydroflumethiazide, cyclothiazide, chlorthiazide

-romycin = Macrolides

Examples: erythromycin, azithromycin, clarithromycin, dirithromycin

Exception: troleandomycin

-phylline = Exanthine derivatives

Examples: theophylline, aminophylline, dyphylline, oxtriphylline

-vir = Antiviral medicines

Examples: acyclovir, cidofovir, ganciclovir, oseltamivir, tenofovir, zanamivir, valganciclovir, valacyclovir

-aine = Local anesthetics

Examples: benzocaine, cocaine, procaine, tetracaine, bupivacaine, etidocaine, lidocaine, etidocaine, mepivacaine, ropivacaine

-bital = Barbiturates

Examples: phenobarbital, mephobarbital

-tyline = Tricyclic antidepressants

Examples: amitriptyline, nortriptyline, protriptyline

Exceptions: amoxapine, clomipramine, despramine, imipramine

-etine = Selective serotonin reuptake inhibitors

Examples: fluoxetine, paroxetine

Exceptions: citalopram, fluvoxamine, sertraline

-quine = Antimalarials

Examples: chloroquine, hydroxychloroquine, mefloquine, primaquin

Exceptions: pyrimethamine, quinine

-acin = Fluoroquinolones

Examples: ciprofloxacin, enoxacin, levofloxacin, norfloxacine

Exception: nalidixic acid

Here are two important prefixes:

sulf- = Sulfa drugs
Examples: sulfadiazine, sulfasalazine, sulfamthizole, sulfisoxazole
Exceptions: mafenide

-ceph- or *cef-* = Cephalosporin
Examples: cefadroxil, cefazolin, cephalexin, cephalothin, cephapirin, cefa-
clor, cefoxitin, cefuroxime, cefixime, cefoperazone, cefotaxime, cef-
prozil, ceftriaxone, cefonicid

*Make it easier to remember by carefully considering the suffix (and prefix)
in the generic name of the medication.*

Remember That the "Marine in Combat" Will Explain the Effects of Sympathetic Nervous System Activation on the Body's Organ Systems

I am convinced that some things never change. With mild amusement, I have
noted the annual ritual of students who are taking the physiology course and
struggling to learn the effects of the sympathetic and parasympathetic
nervous system (autonomic nervous system) on body organs or tissues.

It is so easy to learn if you think of the "Marine in combat."

Does the Marine want to be strong? Of course, so sympathetic stimulation
dilates skeletal muscle arteries and arterioles increasing blood flow to
skeletal muscle. Is blood flow to the skin and internal viscera, for example,
the bowel, essential to promote the safety of the Marine? No, so sympathetic
stimulation constricts skin and visceral vessels, enabling more blood to be
shunted to vital organs.

Does the Marine in combat need to see clearly and as far as possible? Of
course, so sympathetic stimulation dilates the pupils (mydriasis).

Will maximal oxygenation of his lungs be beneficial? Of course, so sympathetic stimulation dilates bronchial smooth muscle increasing tidal volume
and alveolar ventilation.

Does the Marine want to pass urine or have a bowel movement during
combat? Of course not. Thus, sympathetic stimulation relaxes the smooth
muscle in the walls of the bowel and urinary bladder. Further, sympathetic
stimulation causes contraction of the sphincters of the gastrointestinal and
genitourinary tracts.

Will increased cardiac output be beneficial to the Marine? Of course, so
sympathetic stimulation increases heart rate, myocardial contractility, and
ventricular ejection fraction, all resulting in an increase in cardiac output.

Stimulation of the parasympathetic nervous system has opposite effects on organs and tissues. Heart rate slows and cardiac output is lessened; intestinal motility increases and the urinary bladder wall contracts. Bowel and bladder sphincters relax, thus promoting bowel movement and urination.

You must remember:
1. Heightened sympathetic (adrenergic) nervous system activity leads to increased cardiac output, greater physical strength, greater alertness, and improved vision—all to protect the "Marine in combat."
2. Always seek a way to make voluminous information easier to remember.

Remember That Immunoglobulin A (IgA) Is the Primary Antibody That Protects the Body from the Outside World

Immunoglobulins are antibodies that are a primary line of defense against invasion of the body by infectious organisms. They destroy or inactivate attacking organisms by blocking attachment of viruses to cells, by opsonizing bacteria, by activating complement, and by neutralizing protein toxins.

IgA is the immunoglobulin that is the primary defense against infectious organisms in the environment, the "outside world." Thus, IgA is the primary antibody in intestinal mucosa and epithelia in lungs, intestine, breast, genitourinary tracts, and female reproductive tracts. IgA is the primary antibody in external secretions, namely, tears, breast milk, bronchial secretions, vaginal secretions, and intestinal secretions.

In contrast to IgA located in the mucosal secretions, immunoglobulin G and immunoglobulin M are in the bloodstream of the host.

You must remember:
1. IgA is the immunoglobulin in secretions that protect the individual from "outside world" sources of infection.

Chapter 2

The Most Important Word in Diagnosis: *And*

A medical student, bearing a puzzled expression, approached me and related that she had just encountered a patient whose chief complaint was fatigue. The student declared, "I didn't know where to start because so many diseases can cause fatigue." I softly responded, "And." The student was nonplussed; finally, she faintly asked, "What does 'and' mean?"

The practice of medicine is not easy. Despite bountiful advances in investigative technology, the clinician continues to be challenged by the fact that common symptoms may be indicative of disease in many organ systems. Fatigue may be due to anemia, neoplasia, endocrine, cardiovascular, musculoskeletal, and infectious disease. Breathlessness (dyspnea) may result from disorders in the chest, abdomen, nervous system, and psyche.

It is most reassuring when the patient's symptom suggests a specific pathophysiologic mechanism that is confirmed by a physical sign that demonstrates a functional or structural abnormality. For example, a patient has weakness. Physical examination reveals that the apical impulse is in the sixth intercostal space in the anterior axillary line. Weakness *and* a dilated left ventricle that signifies increased ventricular volume (preload) quickly leads to an accurate diagnosis of systolic heart failure (HF).

Unfortunately, not all illnesses are so easily diagnosed. You, as the clinician, must be a medical detective. The detective in a criminal investigation searches for material or chemical evidence. You, the clinician, seek *ands*.

And Is the Most Important Element in Medical Diagnosis

What are some *ands*?

- *And* may link a symptom to a physical examination sign:
  Weakness *and* a dilated left ventricle = systolic heart failure

- *And* may link a symptom to another symptom:
  Sudden weakness of the right arm and leg *and* febrile sweats = endocarditis

- *And* may link a symptom to an abnormal laboratory or imaging result:

    Shortness of breath *and* elevated serum brain natriuretic peptide = heart failure

- *And* may be the link to a geographical location:

    Fever *and* recent global travel to sub-Saharan Africa suggest malaria

Global travel and immigration, increasingly, represent the *And* in the patient whose symptom complex is related to helminth (worm) infection or a zoonotic disease, such as malaria.

The astute clinician must be prepared to use *And* in different pathways. If the symptom does not easily link to a sign in forming the diagnosis, the clinician may start in another direction. For example, in the patient whose symptoms are entirely nonspecific, an abnormal laboratory value often challenges the physician to think "backward" to arrive at the diagnosis.

Let us begin our clinical linkages, our *Ands*.

In the following, *And* links a symptom to a sign.

Fatigue *And*

The patient presenting with weakness and fatigue represents a common, and often perplexing, problem for the clinician. It is because of its many causes that fatigue, an impaired response to effort, represents a challenge. Fatigue may be caused by infectious, cardiac, neoplastic, endocrine, autoimmune, neuromuscular, psychiatric, and pulmonary disorders. But, first, before getting more specific, *the clinician should always think of the patient's medications as the cause of fatigue, or in fact, any symptom!*

1. Fatigue *and* Fever
Any febrile infectious disease may cause transient fatigue. In the patient with persistent fever, consider the following:

- AIDS-related illness
- Endocarditis
- Myxoma in the heart
- Sarcoidosis
- Toxoplasmosis
- Neoplasia, particularly, lymphoma and leukemia

HIV infection leads to CD4 cell depletion and impaired cellular immunity. Ultimately, the immune dysfunction from the HIV type 1 human retrovirus infection leads to the appearance of clinical AIDS. The virus is transmitted sexually and parenterally. Virtually every organ can be involved in this disease. However, the clinician should recognize that fatigue, fever, weight loss, and night sweats are common presenting features.

Toxoplasmosis infects both immunocompetent and immunocompromised patients. Toxoplasma infection in 80% of immunocompetent patients is asymptomatic. When symptomatic, patients most frequently have bilateral, nontender cervical adenopathy. The course of the illness is self-limited. In contrast, immunocompromised patients infected with the protozoan organisms may have encephalitis with headache and confusion, chorioretinitis with eye pain and reduced visual acuity, or pneumonitis with cough and dyspnea.

Sarcoidosis is a disease of unknown etiology that commonly targets the heart, lungs, liver, kidney, eyes, and skin. It is three to four times more common in black patients than white patients. Enlargement of lymph nodes and the parotid gland is frequently noted. The disease most commonly involves the lungs. Thus, initial symptoms of the disease are often pulmonary, for example, cough or dyspnea. The initial radiographic pulmonary involvement is bilateral hilar node enlargement (similar to Hodgkin's disease). As the pulmonary disease progresses, diffuse interstitial fibrosis occurs, causing the patient to have restrictive pulmonary functional impairment. Restrictive lung disease results in hyperventilation resulting in low system $PaCO_2$ and hypoxemia due to impaired transfer of oxygen from alveoli to pulmonary capillaries.

Sarcoidosis may affect any portion of the central or peripheral nervous system. Half of sarcoidosis patients will develop cranial nerve VII palsy. Approximately 75% of patients with untreated sarcoidosis will have elevated serum levels of angiotensin converting enzyme. Calcium metabolism is often abnormal in these patients due to extrarenal production of calcitriol. Hypercalciuria occurs in approximately 50% of cases and hypercalcemia in 10–20%. As a result, nephrocalcinosis and renal failure may occur.

Many neoplasms can present with fever. Hodgkin's disease has a bimodal age distribution, 20 to 30 years and 50 to 60 years. Fever and night sweats are common (20%); these symptoms are less frequently noted in the patient with non-Hodgkin's lymphoma. HIV infection is associated with a fivefold increase in the incidence of Hodgkin's disease.

Renal carcinoma and tumors of the liver (primary and metastatic) are associated frequently with fever. Atrial myxoma is often confused with endocarditis and lymphoma because it may present with fever, malaise, and weight loss. Tumor obstruction at the mitral valve, causing a diastolic murmur, may precipitate pulmonary edema. Additionally, fragments of tumor may cause peripheral embolization or, in the case of a right atrial myxoma, pulmonary embolism.

2. Fatigue *and* Elevated Central Venous Pressure

There are four cardiac disorders associated with fatigue in which the central venous pressure is elevated:

- Right HF resulting from chronic left HF (biventricular failure) due to valvular, hypertensive, or ischemic heart disease
- Pulmonary hypertension due to pulmonary vascular or parenchymal disease
- Cardiac tamponade
- Constrictive pericarditis

The common denominator causing fatigue in these disorders is a reduced cardiac output, particularly, a diminished cardiac output related to effort.

Cardiac tamponade is typically dramatic and is caused by acute pericarditis of any etiology, dissection of the aorta, chest trauma, invasive diagnostic or therapeutic instrumentation, neoplasia, and, rarely, acute myocardial infarction. However, tamponade may be less dramatic, called subacute tamponade, in which the patient slowly develops hemodynamic instability over days, even weeks. These patients generally have fatigue.

The most common cause of constrictive pericarditis in the United States is prior chest irradiation, usually due to lung or breast carcinoma or to lymphoma. The constriction may be clinically evident as early as 3 months after radiotherapy, though the average duration between treatment and hemodynamic constriction is 7 years.

Superior vena cava (SVC) syndrome, due to obstruction of blood flow in the SVC, is increasing in frequency. It usually is caused by thrombosis or external compression of the vein near its entrance into the right atrium. The most common cause of SVC syndrome is malignancy, most notably small cell lung cancer and non-Hodgkin's lymphoma. (Hodgkin's disease rarely is the etiology.) Thrombosis of the vein typically is related to central venous lines attendant to chemotherapy, bone marrow transplantation, parenteral nutrition, and venous access for dialysis. An infectious cause is fibrosing mediastinitis due to histoplasmosis infection. The patient may have dyspnea. Signs include elevated central venous pressure, facial swelling (occasionally with suffusion), and dilated veins on the arms and chest wall.

In the patient younger than 50 years of age whose SVC syndrome etiology is not evident, consider an inherited hypercoagulable state such as Factor V Leiden mutation or prothrombin gene mutation causing venous thrombosis. Antiphospholipid antibody syndrome (APS), causing venous and arterial thrombosis, may be primary or related to systemic lupus erythematosus. APS is suggested in two or more pregnancy losses after 10 weeks of gestation. These hypercoagulable states are important causes of deep vein thrombosis and pulmonary embolism.

Although the central venous pressure is elevated in SVC syndrome, right HF is not present, because right atrial pressure is normal.

3. Fatigue *and* an Apical Impulse That Is Moved to the Left and Downward in the Chest

There are three cardinal determinants of ventricular function, namely, preload, afterload, and contractility. Preload is the volume of blood in a ventricle at end-diastole; thus, preload is *volume dependent*. Afterload is the pressure in the ventricular wall during ejection. Clinically, the two factors that influence left ventricular (LV) afterload are systemic arterial blood pressure and aortic valve stenosis. In each case, the left ventricle must generate increased pressure to eject blood into the aorta. Thus, afterload is *pressure dependent.*

An apical impulse that is moved to the left and downward on the precordium is indicative of LV dilatation that indicates increased preload. Increased preload is found in patients who have chronic mitral regurgitation, chronic aortic regurgitation, and dilated cardiomyopathy. The increased preload and its associated ventricular dilatation leads to systolic heart failure. Systolic HF is physiologically characterized by reduced cardiac output and ejection fraction. The classic symptom related to decreased cardiac output is fatigue/weakness.

In systolic HF, *and* links the symptom (fatigue) to the physical sign (apical impulse displaced to the left and downward) to the pathophysiology (increased preload progressing to decreased LV contractile power) that results in decreased stroke volume and cardiac output. This is systolic HF.

4. Fatigue *and* Ascites

Consider advanced liver disease of any etiology, gastrointestinal or gynecologic malignancy, and constrictive pericarditis. (You now know that constrictive pericarditis is linked to both elevated central venous pressure and ascites.) Right HF always is associated with peripheral edema, but less commonly with ascites. Left HF will not cause congestive hepatomegaly or ascites.

Cirrhosis, with its associated portal hypertension and hypoalbuminemia, is the most common cause of ascites. Ascites in pelvic malignancy is due to peritoneal seeding. Hepatocellular carcinoma and lymphoma, however, may cause ascites without peritoneal metastases. The two most important tests on ascitic fluid are, first, culture and sensitivity, and second, the serum to ascites albumin gradient. A value greater than 1.1 indicates portal hypertension. A gradient less than 1.1 indicates that portal hypertension is not present.

5. Fatigue *and* Petechiae or Purpura

Aplastic anemia, acute leukemia, and in the older male, macroglobulinemia are all characterized by fatigue and petechiae or purpura. Enlargement of the liver and spleen is common in acute leukemia, and blast cells are found upon examination of peripheral blood.

Waldenstrom's macroglobulinemia typically occurs in patients older than 60 years of age. Increased viscosity of blood due to abnormal protein production often causes visual disturbance and impaired consciousness. Lymphadenopathy, splenomegaly, and hepatomegaly are common in these patients.

Fatigue, with Two *Ands*

Fatigue with two *ands*, namely, fatigue *and* fever, and fatigue *and* petechiae, is highly suggestive of infectious endocarditis (IE). The clinical presentation of IE is very variable, depending upon the virulence of the infecting organism, the patient's age, and other important clinical factors, including the presence of indwelling vascular catheters, prosthetic heart valves, and intravenous drug abuse. The patient may appear toxic or chronically ill.

In the more classic expression of the disease, the clinical picture includes fever, night sweats, weakness, dyspnea, and weight loss. A changing heart murmur, petechiae, other skin lesions including Osler's nodes and splinter hemorrhages, and splenomegaly are found in the classic case. Clubbing may not be noted until the infection has been present for 6 weeks. Peripheral manifestations, in addition to stroke and seizure, include emboli to the gut, kidney, and spleen. Elderly patients who have IE commonly have an indolent expression of the disease. In these patients, arthralgia, weakness, low-grade fever, and anemia are more typically found.

Those patients who are infected with a virulent organism, for example, *Staphylococcus aureus*, on the aortic or mitral valve often present with high fever and chills followed by acute destruction of the valve causing acute pulmonary edema. Endocarditis of the tricuspid valve in the intravenous drug abuser is also most commonly due to *Staphylococcus aureus* infection and causes septic pulmonary emboli and lung abscess.

An important clinical note about petechiae:
Petechiae are found in two disorders, thrombocytopenia of any etiology (as in idiopathic thrombocytopenic purpura) and in disorders characterized by the formation of circulating antigen-antibody complexes that are not cleared by the reticuloendothelial system and, thus, deposit in the walls of blood vessels and glomeruli causing a vasculitis. The petechiae in IE result from this vasculitis. (The reticuloendothelial system is composed of phagocytic cells in the lung, spleen, liver, and lymph nodes.)

6. Fatigue *and* Adenopathy

Enlarged lymph nodes, either regional or generalized, may be found in diseases in which fatigue is a prominent symptom. Fatigue and adenopathy suggests one of the following conditions:

- Lymphoma
- Infectious mononucleosis
- Cytomegalovirus infection
- Toxoplasmosis
- Sarcoidosis
- Chronic fatigue syndrome
- Waldenstrom's macroglobulinemia

Despite a sense of marked fatigue, patients with chronic fatigue syndrome have normal muscle strength, and muscle biopsy is normal. Cervical or axillary lymph nodes are typically painful, and biopsy shows reactive hyperplasia.

Patients with infectious mononucleosis have pharyngitis, often with tonsillar exudates, and palatal petechiae. Posterior cervical adenopathy is highly suggestive of this infection. Saliva may remain infectious for 6 months from onset of symptoms. One-third of patients with mononucleosis have superimposed streptococcal tonsillitis that requires antibiotic therapy.

7. Fatigue *and* Hypertension

Antihypertensive medication is the most common cause of fatigue noted by the hypertensive patient. Fatigue and hypertension and hypokalemia suggests hypercortisolism (Cushing's syndrome) or primary hyperaldosteronism (Conn's syndrome). Patients with Cushing's syndrome typically also have round (moon) facies, buffalo hump, and ecchymoses due to easy bruising.

Patients with pheochromocytoma experience fatigue after a paroxysm of palpitation, sweating, tremulousness, and acute hypertension.

8. Fatigue *and* Jaundice

Fatigue is a symptom in the patient who has cholestasis of any etiology, particularly in those diseases associated with intrahepatic jaundice. Acute viral hepatitis is a common cause of fatigue. Primary or metastatic malignancy in the liver must be considered. Primary biliary cirrhosis, typically occurring in the female patient aged 30 to 65 years, is associated with fatigue and itching (and presence of antimitochondrial antibodies in the serum in 95% of cases). Chronic hepatitis, a common cause of fatigue, rarely causes jaundice except in acute cases of hepatic decompensation or end-stage liver disease.

9. Fatigue *and* Hepatosplenomegaly

Diseases to be suspected include acute viral hepatitis, infectious mononucleosis, alcoholic hepatitis, cirrhosis, toxoplasmosis, cytomegalovirus infection, or macroglobulinemia.

10. Fatigue *and* Weight Loss

The clinician should consider malignancy, AIDS-related illness, chronic hepatitis, and apathetic hyperthyroidism in the older patient, that is a patient older than 55 years of age.

Approximately two-thirds of older hyperthyroid patients have the typical symptoms related to increased circulating thyroid hormone, namely, tremulousness, hyperactivity, increased appetite (hyperphagia), and sweating. The remaining patients exhibit decreased appetite (anorexia), weight loss, absence of skin symptoms, and a listless disposition. Atrial fibrillation occurs in approximately 15% of patients who have apathetic hyperthyroidism. An important clinical point: Atrial fibrillation in hyperthyroidism requires anticoagulation because these patients are at significant risk of systemic embolism.

Remember, then, that fatigue and atrial fibrillation in the patient, especially one older than 55 years of age, should make the clinician think of hyperthyroidism.

11. Fatigue *and* Neurologic Signs

Multiple sclerosis, most commonly affecting the patient who is in the third or fourth decade, is associated with fatigue in addition to numbness of the face or hands, extraocular muscle abnormalities, nystagmus, abnormal papillary responses, hyperreflexia, and cerebellar ataxia. Elevated levels of cerebrospinal fluid IgG are found in many patients with multiple sclerosis.

12. Fatigue *and* Cool Skin, Periorbital Edema, Puffiness of the Fingers, and Slow Relaxation of Deep Tendon Reflexes

Fatigue accompanied by this complex of symptoms suggests hypothyroidism, either primary or secondary. Hypothyroidism of any etiology may cause macrocytosis without megaloblastic bone marrow. The most common cause of primary hypothyroidism is chronic autoimmune thyroiditis (Hashimoto's disease). Antithyroid peroxidase enzymes are found in the serum of 90–100% and antithyroglobulin antibodies in 80% of patients. Patients with Hashimoto's disease have an increased risk of developing another autoimmune disease, such as pernicious anemia.

Medications are an important cause of primary hypothyroidism. Lithium can cause goiter and thyroiditis by inhibiting thyroid hormone secretion. Amiodarone, used in the treatment of arrhythmia, has a direct toxic effect on the thyroid gland. The antineoplastic agent sunitinib commonly causes hypothyroidism and may cause a cardiomyopathy with decreased LV ejection fraction and bone marrow suppression.

13. Fatigue *and* Joint Tenderness or Swelling
Fatigue is common in the patient with rheumatoid arthritis who, additionally, has morning stiffness lasting more than 1 hour and bilateral peripheral polyarthritis involving the metacarpophalangeal and proximal interphalangeal joints of the fingers.

14. Fatigue *and* Heart Murmur or Systolic Click
Fatigue is common in the patient who has mitral valve prolapse with a midsystolic click and, commonly, an associated late apical systolic murmur. These patients often have sharp, jabbing noncardiac chest pain, palpitations, and dyspnea.

The rare patient with atrial myxoma typically has fatigue. Examination shows a diastolic murmur that changes in intensity with change in body position. (See the section titled "Fatigue and Fever" earlier in this chapter.)

15. Fatigue *and* Hirsutism and Acne in the Female
Hyperprolactinemia of any etiology is associated with fatigue. Prolactin is secreted only by cells in the pituitary gland. Serum prolactin concentrations increase physiologically during pregnancy.

A pathologic cause of hyperprolactinemia is prolactin cell adenoma of the pituitary gland. In the reproductive-age woman who is not pregnant, the prolactin-secreting adenoma is manifest by oligomenorrhea, infertility, and, infrequently, galactorrhea. The postmenopausal woman, already in a hypogonadal state, is more likely to present with visual disturbance due to the pituitary tumor affecting the optic nerve. In a man, hyperprolactinemia is associated with decreased libido, impotence, and gynecomastia.

Many medicines cause an increase in serum prolactin concentrations. These include risperidone, phenothiazines, haloperidol, metoclopramide, butyrophenones, and domperidone.

16. Fatigue *and* a Normal Physical Examination
The clinician should think of electrolyte imbalance, for example, hyperkalemia, hypokalemia, and hypercalcemia. The physical examination is normal when the serum electrolyte abnormality is mild to moderate; more severe imbalance causes true muscle weakness. Further, marked elevation in serum calcium concentration may cause depression, stupor, and coma.

Important causes of *hypokalemia* include these:

- Respiratory and metabolic alkalosis because potassium leaves the extracellular space and enters cells as hydrogen leaves the cells to enter the circulation in an attempt to normalize pH
- Increased gastrointestinal loss of potassium that occurs with vomiting or diarrhea
- Increased urinary loss of potassium that occurs with loop and thiazide diuretic therapy

It is important to note that both gastrointestinal and urinary loss of potassium are associated with loss of magnesium. In the patient with hypokalemia, the potassium depletion cannot be corrected until the magnesium deficit is reversed.

Electrocardiographic abnormalities of hypokalemia include T wave flattening, increased amplitude of U waves, and ST segment depression. However, there is marked interpatient variability between serum potassium concentration and the electrocardiographic changes.

The most common causes of *hyperkalemia* include acute and chronic renal failure, medications, and adrenal insufficiency. Renal failure leads to hyperkalemia resulting from reduced urinary excretion of potassium. Similarly, angiotensin converting enzyme inhibitors and, less frequently, angiotensin receptor blockers, potassium-sparing diuretics (e.g., spironolactone and triamterene), and nonaspirin, nonsteroidal anti-inflammatory drugs (NSAIDs) cause hyperkalemia resulting from impaired renal excretion of the electrolyte. Adrenal insufficiency produces elevation in serum potassium due to associated mineralocorticoid deficiency in this endocrinopathy.

Hyperkalemia is manifest by progressive electrocardiographic abnormalities, starting with peaked T waves; as serum potassium concentration increases further, a reduction in amplitude of P waves with QRS widening follows; finally, a sine wave and death occur. As in hypokalemia, there is marked interpatient variability between the serum potassium concentration and the electrocardiographic changes.

Hypercalcemia is most commonly due to hyperparathyroidism or neoplastic disease. Cancer causing hypercalcemia may be due to metastases in bone, primary tumors producing paraneoplastic endocrine syndromes in which parathyroid hormone–related proteins are secreted (e.g., ovary, kidney, and lung), multiple myeloma, and lymphoma, occasionally due to calcitriol production. Calcitriol is the active form of vitamin D and promotes renal reabsorption of calcium, increases intestinal absorption of calcium and phosphorus, and promotes calcium and phosphorus mobilization from bone into plasma.

In the following, *and* links the symptom, fatigue, to another symptom.

17. Fatigue *and* Headache

Patients with giant cell arteritis (GCA) commonly have headaches that often are associated with scalp tenderness. (If specifically asked, the patient may relate tenderness of the scalp with brushing or combing of the hair.) The headache may be in the temporal area or generalized. Headache, in conjunction with jaw claudication or acute partial visual impairment, is highly suggestive of GCA. Examination shows temporal artery tenderness and, occasionally, nodularity. (See the section titled "Stroke and Fever," which follows.)

In the following, *and* links the symptom, fatigue, to other symptoms, to signs, and to abnormal laboratory values.

18. Fatigue *and* Anorexia, Weakness, Weight Loss, Lightheadedness upon Arising, Hyperpigmentation of the Skin Creases, Hyponatremia, and Hyperkalemia

In this case, *and* leads to the diagnosis of chronic primary adrenal insufficiency (Addison's disease) that is caused, in most cases, by autoimmune destruction of the adrenal cortex. Infectious causes of this disease include tuberculosis, HIV, and disseminated fungal disease. The adrenal cortical destruction results in a physiologic deficiency in both glucocorticoid and mineralocorticoid hormones. Hyperpigmentation is due to the increased melanocyte-stimulating effect of increased plasma adrenocorticotrophic hormone (ACTH). Orthostatic lightheadedness is noted due to hypovolemia resulting from aldosterone depletion. It is important to recognize that the drop in systolic and diastolic blood pressure upon arising is associated with an increase in heart rate. (In contrast, orthostatic hypotension due to autonomic sympathetic insufficiency is not associated with a compensatory heart rate increase with the drop in blood pressure.) The mineralocorticoid deficiency results in hyponatremia being present in 90% and hyperkalemia in 65% of patients with Addison's disease. Laboratory diagnosis of chronic primary adrenal insufficiency includes abnormally low plasma cortisol and elevated plasma ACTH levels. The cosyntropin test is used to confirm the diagnosis.

Secondary adrenal insufficiency is related to a pituitary disorder, for example, a nonfunctioning pituitary tumor or postradiation or postsurgical effects. Though symptoms are the same as in Addison's disease, hyperpigmentation does not occur, plasma ACTH levels are subnormal, and the serum potassium is normal.

19. Fatigue *and* Arthralgia, Hyperglycemia, and Abnormal Liver Function Tests

In this case, *and* links the symptoms, fatigue and arthralgia, to chemical abnormalities in the body. *And* enables the clinician to recognize that the disease causing this complex is hemochromatosis, an autosomal recessive inherited disease in which there is increased iron absorption in the intestinal tract. The excessive iron is deposited in joints, where it causes arthralgia; in the pancreas, where it causes diabetes mellitus (50% of cases); in the liver, where it causes cirrhosis; in the pituitary gland, where it causes hypogonadism in men; and in the heart, where it causes dilated cardiomyopathy. Close inspection of the skin often reveals a slate gray color, though the hemochromatosis patient is said to have "bronze diabetes."

Let us now move to other clinically important examples of the medical clue called *and*.

Stroke *and* Fever

A former student, now a medical intern, excitedly called me to tell me that one of my clinical aphorisms enabled him to make an important diagnosis that had not been considered by more experienced physicians. A young, previously healthy man had presented with an acute stroke. The cohort of senior physicians was completely puzzled as to the cause of the acute neurologic event. At the time of admission, the patient's temperature was 100.8°F. To his seniors, my former student said, "Stroke and fever equal endocarditis till proven otherwise." Indeed, this impression was confirmed with blood cultures and echocardiography.

Stroke may be caused by thrombotic arterial occlusion, subarachnoid hemorrhage, intracerebral hemorrhage, arteritis, and embolism. Emboli, most commonly arising in the heart, may be noninfected (bland) or infected. Infected vegetations on heart valves produce the cardiogenic emboli in endocarditis.

The important clinical point is that stroke and fever equal endocarditis (till proven otherwise). Patients who present with an acute stroke and are febrile must be considered as having endocarditis. Obtaining blood cultures and performing echocardiographic imaging are essential.

In infective endocarditis, bacteremia is complicated by development of vegetations that deposit on heart valves or congenital cardiac and vascular anomalies, for example, ventricular septal defect and coarctation of the aorta. The virulence of the infecting organism determines the clinical presentation of the patient. Virulent organisms such as *Staphylococcus aureus* cause the patient to become acutely ill and present with high fever, night sweats, and rapid and severe destruction of a heart valve, which causes regurgitation. Endocarditis resulting from infection with commensal organisms of the mouth and pharynx, for example, *Streptococcus viridans*, presents in a more insidious (subacute) character, often manifest by low-grade fever, anorexia, and arthralgia. In subacute disease, fever is low grade (< 102.5°F) and not associated with chills.

The signs associated with endocarditis involve the heart, skin, central nervous system, eye, joints, and kidney. A new or changing heart murmur is heard in approximately 80% of cases. The murmur may not be loud. Endocarditis of the tricuspid valve may not produce an audible murmur. Skin manifestations include Janeway lesions, painless and erythematous macules, and papules on the palms and soles that represent septic emboli. Petechiae, Osler's nodes (painful, violaceous nodules on the fleshy part of the toes and fingers), and splinter hemorrhages represent deposition of circulating immune complexes. Septic emboli are common because the infected valvular vegetations are friable. In addition to emboli to the brain, the first manifestation of endocarditis is often an embolus to the kidney, spleen, and with right-sided endocarditis, the lung. Tricuspid valve endocarditis, particularly common in intravenous drug abusers, causes suppurative pulmonary emboli and lung abscess formation.

Another important clinical point is not well recognized in patients who have endocarditis. Patients who have been successfully treated for the cardiac infection are at risk of suffering another type of stroke, a subarachnoid hemorrhage, due to rupture of a mycotic aneurysm. A mycotic aneurysm is a weakening and ballooning of an artery due to endocarditis-related infection in the wall of that vessel. The aneurysm in the brain may rupture weeks or even months after the end of antibiotic therapy.

In contrast to endocarditis, an important clinical point: Patients who have occlusive arterial thrombotic stroke, bland (noninfected) cerebral emboli, subarachnoid hemorrhage, and intracerebral hemorrhage *are not febrile at the time of symptom onset.* Fever may be initially noted a day or two after the vascular insult due to a "stress" response. In this case, the fever spontaneously subsides in a few days. However, fever appearing after a stroke should raise strong suspicion of secondary infection occurring in the urinary tract or lung, or infection arising at an intravenous access site. Interestingly, it is very uncommon for an acute, noninfected thrombotic stroke to present with seizure. If seizure is the presenting manifestation, a cerebral embolus or subarachnoid hemorrhage is most likely. However, seizures are very common after stroke (starting at least 2 weeks after the acute event) and account for 50% of epilepsy in older adults.

One disease closely mimics endocarditis. In fact, this condition may also present with stroke and fever. I refer to GCA. GCA is a vasculitis that affects branches of the external carotid artery, yet may involve other arteries arising from the aorta. It is a disease that affects persons older than 50 years of age;

the average age at time of onset is 70 years. GCA is not a rare disorder; the prevalence is considered to be 200 per 100,000 adults. Although GCA is not rare, the problem is that it is rarely diagnosed.

Onset of GCA symptoms may be gradual or abrupt. Systemic symptoms that mimic endocarditis include fever in 50% of cases, even spiking to 104°F, fatigue, and weight loss. Both infectious endocarditis and GCA may present with stroke and fever.

Symptoms related to narrowing or occlusion of cranial arteries that are more specific to GCA and not endocarditis include headache with temporal artery tenderness, jaw claudication (50% of cases), abrupt partial visual defect that may be transient (amaurosis fugax) or permanent, arm claudication, and polymyalgia rheumatica (PMR). Jaw claudication is caused by ischemia of the masseter muscles and is characterized by aching in the jaw with chewing. Symptoms disappear in a few minutes when chewing is discontinued.

PMR is characterized by symmetrical aching and morning stiffness in the shoulders, hip girdle, neck, and torso. It occurs in half of patients who have GCA. There is no specific laboratory test that defines GCA. The erythrocyte sedimentation rate (ESR) is usually very high, greater than 90 mm/hr, yet may be normal in 4% of cases. (The ESR in endocarditis would expectedly be elevated, but not nearly approaching levels seen in GCA.) Other common laboratory abnormalities include normochromic anemia with normal leukocyte count, increased platelet count, abnormal serum alkaline phosphatase and aminotransferase, and elevated serum C-reactive protein. GCA diagnosis is confirmed by temporal artery biopsy.

The bottom line is that any patient presenting with a stroke must have an accurate temperature measurement and ESR determination. Blood cultures must be obtained if fever is present.

Please note that diseases present with fever and acute neurologic deterioration that are not strokes. These include encephalitis, meningitis, subdural empyema, and brain abscess. Encephalitis is most commonly of viral origin; meningitis may be caused by many classes of infectious agents. Brain abscess occurs from hematogenous spread of infection from other sites in the body, such as gums or skin, or from trauma as may occur in a bullet wound in the head.

Heart Failure *and* Bounding Pulses

HF is a broad umbrella diagnosis that includes disorders with varied pathophysiology, symptoms, physical signs, and treatment. Systolic HF, for example, is characterized by weakness, dilated left ventricle, and reduced cardiac output. Diastolic HF (DHF) is characterized by dyspnea and a non-compliant left ventricle.

In the patient who has HF manifest by dyspnea, peripheral edema, gallop heart rhythm, and pulmonary crackles, and in whom examination shows bounding arterial pulses, the clinician should immediately exclude the diagnoses of systolic HF and DHF. Rather, the clinician should consider high cardiac output HF. The bounding pulses are associated with increased pulse pressure, systolic hypertension, and tachycardia, all related to decreased peripheral (systemic) vascular resistance and increased stroke volume. HF and bounding pulses are characteristic of hyperthyroidism, arteriovenous fistula, and beri beri.

Hyperthyroidism may result from an autoimmune disease (Graves' disease) in which anti-thyroid stimulating hormone receptor antibodies are present in the serum. These antibodies *stimulate* thyroid hormone synthesis, in contrast to autoimmune antibodies in other diseases that have an antagonistic effect upon the receptor organ. Other nonautoimmune causes of hyperthyroidism include toxic adenoma, toxic multinodular goiter, exogenous intake of thyroid hormone, and, causing a transient hyperthyroid state, thyroiditis.

Arteriovenous fistulas may be congenital or, more commonly, acquired. Acquired causes include surgical construction of a fistula for vascular access in patients requiring chronic hemodialysis and those patients who have suffered penetrating wounds, usually from a bullet or stabbing. Again, the bounding pulses are a result of the decreased systemic vascular resistance in these patients. Interestingly, HF from a penetrating wound tends to occur about 2 years after the injury, but may occur, infrequently, as early as 6 months after injury. High cardiac output HF in thiamine deficiency is called "wet beri beri." The *wet* form of beri beri due to vitamin B thiamine deficiency is more common in Asian countries in which the population ingests a diet high in polished rice (and low in thiamine).

In contrast to high output HF with its wide pulse pressure due to increased stroke volume in the presence of low systemic vascular resistance, many persons have increased pulse pressure related to an entirely different mechanism. Pulse pressure is simply the difference between systolic and diastolic blood pressure. Increased stiffness (or decreased compliance) of large arteries results in an increased systolic pressure during LV ejection. Then, during ventricular diastole, the reduced elasticity in the stiff aorta results in a decrease in diastolic pressure. As a result, elderly persons commonly have increased pulse pressure yet do not have the hemodynamic abnormalities, for example, increased stroke volume and low systemic vascular resistance, that are noted in high cardiac output states.

Dyspnea *And*

Dyspnea (breathlessness) is a common symptom that may be mild in character or may create fear of impending death. Of course, as in the case of many symptoms, there are many causes, including cardiac, pulmonary, musculoskeletal, neurologic, and psychiatric disorders. In the majority of patients with dyspnea, the etiology is lung disease or heart disease; so-called pulmonary dyspnea and cardiac dyspnea.

In many patients, clinical experience has taught me a very simple *and* that can help differentiate between these two disorders. *And* is the link between the symptom, dyspnea, and *the location of the point of maximal impulse (PMI)* on the precordium. The clinical principle: If the PMI is a lift or heave at the apex, think of cardiac dyspnea. If the PMI is a lift along the left sternal border, think of pulmonary dyspnea.

Let us explore the basis of this clinical point. The pathophysiology in *pulmonary dyspnea* is complex. The normal pulmonary artery pressure in the adult at rest is approximately 24/9 with a mean of 15 mm Hg. Pulmonary hypertension is defined as a mean pulmonary artery pressure greater than 25 mm Hg at rest. In those patients in whom increased pulmonary vascular resistance occurs, for example, in those with interstitial lung disease (pulmonary fibrosis), chronic bronchitis, hypoxemia and alveolar ventilation from thoracovertebral deformities, and pulmonary embolic disease, pulmonary hypertension follows.

The increased pulmonary artery pressure increases right ventricular pressure designed to preserve cardiac output. In turn, increased right ventricular pressure causes both right ventricular dilatation and hypertrophy. The clinical sign is a left parasternal lift. Therefore, if the dyspneic patient has a left parasternal lift as the PMI, the clinician knows that pulmonary hypertension is present.

The common denominator in cardiac dyspnea is an increase in left atrial mean pressure. The elevated left atrial pressure is transmitted retrograde through the pulmonary veins into the pulmonary capillaries. The lungs become stiff due to pulmonary congestion, that is, interstitial edema, and the patient experiences breathlessness. DHF is the classic cardiac disorder causing dyspnea.

Let's look closely at *cardiac dyspnea* associated with DHF. DHF is due to increased stiffness (decreased compliance) of the left ventricle. The stiff ventricle has an elevated end-diastolic pressure. Therefore, left atrial pressure must increase in an effort to propel blood forward into the ventricle during diastole. Again, this elevated left atrial pressure is transmitted backward into the lungs, causing dyspnea. DHF is most commonly associated with left ventricular hypertrophy (LVH). LVH, in turn, is a compensatory response to systemic hypertension or aortic valve stenosis. The physical sign of LVH is an apical lift or heave and, if the patient is in sinus rhythm, an S4 gallop. LVH, then, may be *acquired*, secondary to hypertension or aortic valve stenosis, or LVH may be *related to congenital heart disease*, for example, hypertrophic cardiomyopathy.

Increased LV stiffness may be due to factors other than hypertrophy. Myocardial ischemia commonly is associated with *transiently increased stiffness*. This explains why the patient, during an attack of angina pectoris, often has associated breathlessness. After sublingual nitroglycerin use, the angina disappears and the dyspnea disappears. Further, the transient myocardial ischemia–induced stiffness of the LV explains "anginal equivalent" in which the patient has dyspnea due to transient DHF, but the patient has no associated anginal discomfort. Another cause of increased LV stiffness that can present as DHF is infiltrative myocardial disease, for example, amyloidosis.

Clubbing *And*

It is most important to recognize that clubbing of fingers and toes is not a sign of chronic obstructive pulmonary disease (COPD). If a patient with COPD develops clubbing, a careful search for another cause, especially lung cancer, must be made.

Clubbing is associated with many conditions, including primary and metastatic lung cancer, cyanotic congenital heart disease, infective endocarditis, nonmalignant pulmonary disease, cirrhosis, and inflammatory bowel disease. Clubbing may be familial and present without an associated disease.

Further, there is a related condition, hypertrophic osteoarthropathy (HO), a painful disorder in which there is subperiosteal formation of new bone. This causes pain in knees, ankles, shoulders, elbows, and wrists. HO is found in patients whose clubbing is associated with lung cancer (most commonly adenocarcinoma and least commonly with small cell carcinoma), mesothelioma, cirrhosis, and bronchiectasis.

The clinician must make the link between the clubbing and other clinical features. Here are some examples:

1. Clubbing *and* Recurrent Pulmonary Infections

Clubbing and recurrent pulmonary infections in a noncyanotic child suggests cystic fibrosis (CF). CF is an autosomal recessive hereditable disease that is the most common cause of chronic lung disease in children and young adults. It is a disorder that affects all exocrine glands with production of viscous secretions in the respiratory, gastrointestinal, and reproductive tracts. Pulmonary involvement includes chronic bronchitis, bronchiectasis, and cor pulmonale. Pancreatic insufficiency and infertility are common. The majority of CF patients have sinus disease and nasal polyps. *Pseudomonas* infection is responsible for the majority of deaths in patients.

A common complication of CF is bronchiectasis manifest by long-standing cough, mucopurulent sputum production, wheezing, and, occasionally, hemoptysis, even massive in quantity. Bronchiectasis may occur in patients who do not have CF. Non-CF bronchiectasis is related to airway obstruction due to a foreign body in the lung (even unchewed food from aspiration), repeated pulmonary infection, presumably due to viral or mycoplasma infection, and allergic bronchopulmonary aspergillosis that may occur in the long-standing asthmatic patient. In non-CF bronchiectasis, the incidence of clubbing is directly related to the severity of the pulmonary disorder.

An important clinical point: Up to 7% of CF patients are initially diagnosed at the age of 18 years or older.

2. Clubbing *and* Lung Abscess

Lung abscess is most commonly related to two conditions, aspiration and septic embolism to the lung from tricuspid endocarditis. Lung abscess is characterized by cough, purulent (often foul-smelling) sputum, fever, and night sweats. In aspiration, the most common infecting organisms are anaerobic bacteria that are normally found in gingival crevices. These include *Peptostreptococcus*, *Bacteroides* spp, and *Fusobacterium*.

Aspiration occurs in patients predisposed to impaired consciousness, for example, those suffering from chronic alcohol or drug abuse or those who have a seizure disorder. These patients are prone to vomiting, during which time the vomitus carries gingival organisms into the lungs. The pulmonary infection typically causes abscess formation in 7 to 14 days.

It is important to recognize that, in the patient with lung abscess due to aspiration, sputum cultures and even bronchoscopy specimens are contaminated by upper airway flora. Therefore, in this patient a transtracheal aspirate is essential to obtain a sputum sample that will correctly identify the infecting organism in the lungs.

Intravenous drug abusers commonly develop lung abscess secondary to septic emboli from tricuspid endocarditis. In fact, three-quarters of patients with tricuspid endocarditis have septic emboli to the lungs. The infecting organism is most commonly *Staphylococcus aureus*. This virulent organism causes the patient to be toxic, exhibiting high fever, chills, and night sweats. The classic murmur of tricuspid regurgitation is a holosystolic murmur in the fourth intercostal space that increases during inspiration. However, in many patients with tricuspid endocarditis, a murmur may not be heard on auscultation.

3. Clubbing *and* Cyanotic Congenital Heart Disease

Clubbing is common in cyanotic congenital heart diseases such as tetralogy of Fallot and transposition of the great arteries. In most cases, arterial desaturation must be present for at least 6 months before clubbing is evident. However, in severe cases clubbing may be noted at 3 months of age. In tetralogy, a right-sided aortic arch is present in approximately 25% of cases.

Clubbing and cyanosis are characteristic in patients who have Eisenmenger syndrome. Those who are born with noncyanotic congenital heart disease with large left to right shunts, as may occur in atrial septal defect, ventricular septal defect, and patent ductus arteriosus, are at risk of developing Eisenmenger syndrome. The pathophysiologic abnormality in this syndrome is development of increased pulmonary vascular resistance with resultant pulmonary hypertension that causes *reversal of shunt direction*. Patients then have right to left shunting that causes severe systemic arterial desaturation and clubbing formation.

4. Clubbing *and* Pulmonary Fibrosis (Interstitial Lung Disease)

Pulmonary fibrosis may be idiopathic or due to environmental disorders or to medication. Inorganic (silicon dioxide) and organic dusts (avian antigens), fumes (chlorine, isocyanates), and medications (for example, amiodarone, sulfonamides, phenytoin, cyclophosphamide, and methotrexate) are recognized agents that incite the pulmonary inflammatory process.

The pathophysiologic common denominators are decreased pulmonary compliance (or increased lung stiffness) that causes a restrictive pulmonary disorder in addition to impairment of oxygen transfer from the alveoli to the pulmonary capillaries. Restrictive lung disease is characterized by hyperventilation (without airway obstruction), hypocapnia (low $PaCO_2$), and variable hypoxemia (low PaO_2) dependent upon severity of the disease. Chest radiography shows reticulonodular infiltrates most pronounced in the lower lung fields. Clubbing occurs in 25% to 50% of patients who have pulmonary fibrosis. Pulmonary function tests in the patient with restrictive lung disease show a normal or increased forced expiratory volume 1 sec/forced vital capacity ratio (FEV 1 sec/FVC), decreased carbon monoxide diffusing capacity, and reduced tidal volume. In contrast, the FEV 1 sec/FVC ratio is reduced in patients having obstructive airway disease, such as asthma and chronic bronchitis.

Hyperglycemia *And*

A number of diseases cause hyperglycemia and cause secondary diabetes mellitus. The clinician must look for the *and* that links the elevated plasma glucose to the correct etiology.

1. Hyperglycemia *and* obesity, hirsutism, oligomenorrhea (or amenorrhea), and infertility is characteristic of polycystic ovary syndrome (PCO). PCO is associated with insulin resistance and hyperinsulinemia that frequently leads to type 2 diabetes mellitus. In addition to hyperglycemia, PCO patients have increased serum levels of luteinizing hormone, testosterone, and prolactin. Because of increased androgen levels, the patients have a male hair distribution.

2. Hyperglycemia *and* hypertension in a patient who has a rounded ("moon") facies and ecchymoses is indicative of hypercortisolemia. The elevated serum cortisol levels may be due to a functioning pituitary adenoma (Cushing's disease), adrenal hyperplasia or carcinoma, or to glucocorticoid medicinal therapy. Hyperglycemia is present because cortisol (and glucocorticoid medication) increases gluconeogenesis and inhibits glycogen storage.

3. Hyperglycemia *and* slowly enlarging jaw, hands, and feet in an adult patient is typical of acromegaly. Acromegaly is caused by a pituitary adenoma that secretes elevated levels of growth hormone and prolactin. Growth hormone stimulates glucagon release. As a result, insulin resistance and hyperinsulinemia are noted in 60% of patients; another 15% have diabetes mellitus. Hypertension is common, present in 50% of acromegalic patients.

    Think for a moment: Note how you can reverse the clues in the preceding two patients. Start with hypertension and add the physical signs as *and*. Now you have "hypertension *and*": Hypertension *and* a moon facies suggests hypercortisolemia. Hypertension *and* enlarging hands and feet is indicative of acromegaly.

4. Hyperglycemia *and* episodic sweats, palpitations, and headache suggests pheochromocytoma. Pheochromocytomas are tumors that secrete excessive amounts of norepinephrine or epinephrine. Most patients have

sustained hypertension; a small percentage (5–15%) have normal blood pressure with paroxysmal elevations. The hyperglycemia is due to an increase in both hepatic glycogenolysis and gluconeogenesis. Those patients with sustained hypertension often have superimposed *orthostatic hypotension* due to the hypovolemia induced by chronic elevation in plasma catecholamines. Diagnosis is made by urine assays that show increased excretion of metanephrines and catecholamines.

Approximately 15% of pheochromocytomas occur as hereditable disorders. Both have autosomal dominant inheritance. First is von Hippel–Lindau syndrome characterized by pheochromocytoma, retinal angioma, cerebellar hemangioblastoma, renal and pancreatic cysts, and renal carcinoma. The second is multiple endocrine neoplasia type 2 A (MEN 2A). In this condition the pheochromocytoma is often associated with medullary carcinoma of the thyroid and parathyroid hyperplasia that cause hyperparathyroidism.

5. Hyperglycemia *and* flushing and diarrhea suggests medullary carcinoma of the thyroid. This neuroendocrine tumor is usually sporadic; approximately 15% are part of multiple endocrine neoplasia type 2 (MEN 2) syndrome. The tumors usually secrete several chemicals, particularly calcitonin, but also serotonin, prostaglandins, and adrenocorticotrophic hormone (ACTH). The hypercortisolism induced by ACTH causes hyperglycemia in these tumors.

6. Hyperglycemia *and* azotemia. Most commonly, patients with type 1 and type 2 diabetes mellitus develop hypertension with progressive renal involvement associated with the endocrine disorder. In the type 1 diabetic, blood pressure typically begins to rise within 3 years of the onset of microalbuminuria. In the type 2 diabetic, hypertension is common prior to presence of microalbuminuria. In these patients, obesity is common, and the hypertension is likely due to the patient's weight. The mechanism by which obesity increases blood pressure is not clear. Persistent obesity not only increases blood pressure, but makes the condition more difficult to control by interfering with the effect of anti-hypertensive medication.

7. Hyperglycemia *and* acanthosis nigricans (AN) is a clinical disorder indicative of the insulin resistance found in all patients who have *non-malignancy*-associated AN. AN is found in diabetes mellitus, obesity, and Cushing's syndrome.

Further, AN is associated with *malignancy*, especially gastric and hepatocellular carcinoma and less frequently lung cancer. AN lesions are gray-brown to black, are rough in texture, and are most commonly found in the axillae, inguinal creases, and back and sides of the neck.

Eosinophilia *And*

Eosinophilia, defined as more than 500 eosinophiles/microL, is common in allergic (atopic) disorders such as allergic rhinitis and asthma. Diagnosis is usually quite easy. In rhinitis the *nasal secretions* demonstrate eosinophiles upon Gram stain examination. Further, in asthma the *sputum secretions* contain eosinophiles; this can be helpful in differentiation from chronic obstructive lung disease.

Eosinophilia is also noted in certain acute leukemias and neoplasms, for example, in 15% of patients with Hodgkin's lymphoma. Eosinophilia is noted in 20% of patients with systemic mastocytosis, a neoplastic disorder in which mast cells accumulate in skin, liver, spleen, bone marrow, and lymph nodes. Symptoms arise when mast cells release histamine, leukotrienes, heparin, and prostaglandins. Hypotension, flushing, diarrhea, and pruritus are typical manifestations.

Eosinphilia also may result from ingestion of many medications. Examples include NSAIDs, beta adrenergic blockers, phenytoin, cephalosporins, and the histamine H2 receptor antagonist ranitidine.

In the preceding disorders, the clinician has a clear indication of the etiology of the increased eosinophile blood count. However, there are many times, after performing a history and physical examination, when the clinician cannot determine the diagnosis. At these times, the eosinophilia may be the seminal clue in the clinical puzzle. The abnormal laboratory result may coax the clinician to search for another *and*. In the case of eosinophilia, *and* often represents international travel. Of course, international travel relates both to the immigrant as well as to the American who travels abroad, becomes infected, and then returns.

Many helminth (worm) parasitic diseases cause eosinophilia; the degree is related to the extent of parasitic invasion of the intestinal mucosa. Parasitic worms that cause human infection include nematodes (roundworms), cestodes (tapeworms), and trematodes (flukes). Trichinellosis, a nematode infection, is common in East Asia and South America. Moreover, it is not rare in the United States because human infection may be acquired by ingestion of *Trichinella* cysts from inadequately cooked pork from domestic pigs.

In trichinellosis, invasion of the intestinal mucosa causes abdominal discomfort, nausea, vomiting, and diarrhea. Hematogenous spread of the larvae to skeletal muscle follows. Muscle pain occurs; at this point, the patient has muscle tenderness, splinter and conjunctival hemorrhages, periorbital edema, and chemosis. Eosinophilia appears approximately 1 week after the onset of muscle symptoms.

Conclusion

A patient's symptom guides the clinician's thinking toward diagnosis. It is *and* that enables the astute medical detective to quickly sort through the differential diagnosis to reach an efficient and correct diagnosis.

Always seek the *and* when searching for diagnosis.

Chapter 3

MED1C and a Word on Drug Interactions

MED1C

Advances in pharmacology have significantly reduced the mortality and morbidity of infectious diseases. As in all things, unintended consequences have attended the explosive growth in the pharmacopoeia. Illustrative is antibiotic resistance related to the profligate use of antimicrobial agents. Certainly, all students in the health professions are cautioned that every drug may have adverse effects.

Despite the tocsin—the warning—that a medicine may cause illness rather than alleviate it, experienced clinicians regrettably are unaware that medicines are an extremely common *and unrecognized* cause of symptoms and illness in patients.

Basic Precepts in Medical Practice

Over decades in medical practice, the most fundamental precept that I have learned is that the most important element in medical care is a caring attitude. I suggest that *MED1C* is a close second in importance.

The MED1C acronym means "*MED*icine" is the number *1* Consideration in all patient encounters. Let me be clear: *Medicine* not only includes prescribed medication, but also over-the-counter medical preparations, vitamins, nose sprays, and alternative and complementary products.

MED1C directs that you must remember these points:

- When a patient has a new *symptom*, think first of medication as the etiology.
- When a patient demonstrates a new *abnormal sign upon physical examination*, think first of medication as the cause.
- When the patient's evaluation reveals a new *abnormal laboratory value or imaging abnormality*, think first of medication as the etiology.

The medication may be taken presently, recently, or in unusual cases in the distant past.

Clinical Vignettes and MED1C

The following clinical vignettes illustrate how MED1C led to quick and correct diagnosis of an apparently confusing medical illness.

Clinical Vignette, Patient A: "My Husband Is Dying of Cancer. . . . But They Can't Find It."

It occurred many years ago when I thought of myself as a well-trained but still inchoate physician. I entered an examining room to see a patient, a dear lady distressed by the physical limitations imposed by chronic heart failure.

I noticed another woman seated in the small room. After a warm hug, my patient introduced me to her sister who was visiting from New Jersey. Following a brief, respectful greeting, I began to ask my patient of her present symptoms. It was only seconds before the sister began to weep almost inaudibly. "Why are you crying?" Softly, she responded, "My husband is dying of cancer." I expressed regret and, again, turned to my patient.

"But they can't find it." Once more, I turned to the sister and repeated in disbelief, "Your husband is dying of cancer, but they can't find it?"

"Yes, he has lost 35 pounds, is profoundly weak—and every test is normal. The doctors say he must have cancer."

I had been counseled by older physicians to "not get involved" in medical problems of those who were not my patients. Yet, impulsively, I asked whether the husband was taking a then commonly prescribed (now off the market) hypnotic agent. "Yes, every night." I stated that I had read a report that this hypnotic could, in rare cases, cause marked weight loss and weakness. I volunteered the gentle suggestion that she speak to her husband's physician and inquire whether the sleeping pill might be discontinued.

Three weeks later, I received a call from New Jersey. "The medicine was stopped. The cancer is gone. My husband has gained 7 pounds and he is feeling stronger."

The "malignancy" was cured by simply recognizing that the patient's profound distress was an adverse effect of the medicine.

Clinical Vignette, Patient B: The Intractable Headaches

In south Florida, we physicians have many "snowbird" patients. These are patients whose permanent homes are in the north, but who sojourn in our warm, sunny climate during the winter months.

Once frost had returned to Ontario Province, Canada, my snowbird patient was back to see me. Intelligent, sophisticated, a man of probity, and affluent. How could I not remember that he owned a Rolls Royce Phantom? At his first visit, he was obviously in distress. For nearly 2 months he had suffered intractable, diffuse headaches, only relieved by potent analgesics. A consultant in neurology could find no cause. Computerized tomography and magnetic resonance imaging studies were normal. The decision was made to continue the analgesics, but if the headaches persisted, he would undergo cerebral angiography when he returned to Canada.

I had always taught my patients to bring a written list of medications when they came in for a medical visit. After speaking of the headaches, my patient dutifully handed me his list. Immediately, I noted that he was taking a hypnotic that I knew could cause headaches. "I'll bet you a nickel that your headaches will go away if you stop this medicine." Immediately heartened by a positive word, my patient took my hand. The handshake sealed the bet.

Ten days later, the patient returned with a broad grin. Happily, the headaches had ceased. The patient placed a coin in my hand. Standing at the window in my office where I could look down upon the parked Phantom, I realized that my grateful patient had paid his debt with a Canadian nickel, 3.8 cents U.S.

Clinical Vignette, Patient C: Flushing and the Professor's Mother

It was a delight to care for this elderly lady. She was an octogenarian, still vibrant and full of inquisitive energy. She was much too special to label as a "snowbird," though she was another 4-month-per-annum patient. Her son was a professor in an illustrious northeastern medical school.

My patient told me that she had for several months experienced frequent and distressing episodes of flushing and sweats. At her son's direction, a medical colleague had carried out extensive diagnostic testing, including urinary studies for catecholamines (pheochromocytoma) and 5-hydroxytryptamine (carcinoid syndrome) in addition to serum calcitonin concentration (medullary carcinoma of the thyroid).

The patient had had no menopausal symptoms for years; therefore, she was not experiencing hot flashes. She drank no alcohol, and there were no skin lesions to suggest mastocytosis. Naturally, I asked of her medicine intake. Moreover, I specifically inquired about intake of vitamins, use of any nose sprays, or ingestion of medicinal herbs or roots.

I was surprised when she told me of niacin vitamin intake. "Didn't the physician at the medical school ask you about medicines?"

"He did, but vitamins are not medicines, so I didn't tell him."

The troubling flushes were immediately cured with cessation of niacin intake.

Clinical Vignette, Patient D: The Student, Not the Physician, Makes the Medical Diagnosis

A medical student experiences the insidious onset of malaise and fatigue, nausea, anorexia, and dark (tea-colored) urine. His visit to a medical clinic quickly led to a diagnosis of acute hepatitis. All serologic tests for antibodies to hepatitis viruses were negative. The physician told the student that he "must have viral hepatitis but I can't prove it."

The patient had a friend, a physician assistant student, who had learned MED1C in my class. Upon inquiry of medicines presently or recently taken, the hepatitis patient said that 2 weeks earlier he had taken an erythromycin preparation for bronchitis.

The patient had an adverse reaction that caused a chemical hepatitis. Overall, statistics suggest that drug hepatotoxicity accounts for nearly 10% of cases of acute hepatitis in adults and approximately 40% of cases in patients over the age of 50 years.

One more vignette that signifies the subtlety of MED1C.

Clinical Vignette, Patient E: The Unusual Manifestations of Thyroid Hormone Therapy

A 64-year-old woman began to note that her dreams were much more "active"; they were not violent in character, but voices of persons speaking in the dreams were louder and movement was much faster. These dreams were distressing to the patient and kept her from restful sleep. At the same time, she began to note aching in teeth and gums. The patient consulted her dentist, who found no evidence of infection or cavity. Rather, he strongly suspected that the patient had begun to have involuntary jaw clenching that was causing the gingival and tooth discomfort.

A puzzling pair of symptoms—mouth aching and dynamic dreams. The patient's husband, a physician, asked whether there was any change in medication intake. Indeed, her endocrinologist had minimally increased the dosage of levothyroxine hormone in treatment of mild hypothyroidism.

The patient called her physician and asked whether dosage could be reduced to the earlier level. Three weeks after return to the previous dosage, her dreams were more relaxed and the jaw clenching–induced tooth and gum aching had ended.

Abnormal Laboratory Values and MED1C

Let us turn to abnormal laboratory values and MED1C. Here are three examples.

MED1C and Liver Function Tests

Many medications are hepatotoxic: those that cause hepatocellular necrosis with elevation of serum aminotransferase levels and those that primarily cause cholestasis with subsequent elevation of serum gamma glutamyl transpeptidase and alkaline phosphatase. There are three mechanisms of liver injury:

- Intrinsic hepatotoxins, for example, carbon tetrachloride or acetaminophen (large doses)
- Hypersensitivity reaction, for example, halothane, sulfonamides
- Abnormal metabolism of the medication that leads to cell necrosis

MED1C and Plasma Glucose Level

Often, the clinician notes that a patient has elevation of plasma glucose. Remember that hyperglycemia may be caused by several medications:

- Niacin
- Prednisone and other glucocorticoids
- Thiazides and loop diuretics

MED1C and Serum Creatinine

The serum creatinine value is important in estimating renal function and glomerular filtration rate. The clinician must be aware that the antibiotic trimethoprim sulfamethoxazole and the H2-blocker cimetidine are commonly prescribed medications that decrease renal secretion of creatinine and thus cause a reversible increase in serum values as much as 0.4 to 0.5 mg/dL. Famotidine and ranitidine can also increase serum creatinine values, but to a lesser degree. Note that these medications do not increase the blood urea nitrogen value. Only if an increase in serum creatinine value is accompanied by a corresponding increase in blood urea nitrogen is there a true decrease in glomerular filtration rate.

Here are a few examples of medication-induced disorders that will reinforce MED1C.

- Acute pericarditis caused by isoniazid hydrazide (INH): Taken by the patient who has latent tuberculosis infection, for example, INH may precipitate acute pericardial inflammation. Any medication that has a hydrazide chemical radical can cause acute pericarditis, for example, hydralazine.

- Goiter in the patient who takes lithium therapy: Lithium inhibits thyroid hormone secretion. The reduced serum levels of thyroid hormone lead to increased pituitary secretion of thyroid stimulating hormone (TSH). In turn, elevated serum TSH causes diffuse, nonnodular thyroid enlargement (goiter). Approximately 50% of lithium-treated patients have goiter.

- Left ventricular (LV) dilation in the patient who takes chemotherapy: The anthracycline class of chemotherapy agents is cardiotoxic. One of these, doxorubicin, can cause LV dilation, reduced ejection fraction, and systolic heart failure.

When the Clinician Does Not Remember MED1C

The clinician who does not remember MED1C is likely to fall into the trap called "cascading" of drugs. Cascading means that an additional medicine is prescribed for a new medical condition caused by present medicine intake.

I remember the classic example of cascading that occurred years ago when I was a resident in medicine. A patient was seen in the medical clinic for treatment of heart failure. Review of the medical record indicated that the patient, initially, had hypertension for which a thiazide diuretic was prescribed. Subsequently, hyperuricemia and urate kidney stones developed. Physicians in the urology clinic were reluctant to discontinue a drug prescribed in another clinic. Therefore, thiazide therapy was continued and, also, sodium bicarbonate was prescribed in an effort to alkalinize the urine to dissolve existing stones and prevent formation of new ones. Perhaps not unexpectedly, the patient developed dyspnea and heart failure for which digoxin therapy was added to his diuretic regimen.

Clearly, the first step in proper care of the patient would have been discontinuation of the thiazide diuretic. Alas, in this case, the thiazide was not stopped. Rather, a cascade of medicines was prescribed in treatment of the medical problems caused by the thiazide.

Cascading continues in contemporary medicine. Examples include initiation of antihypertensive therapy in the patient who develops hypertension from nonaspirin, nonsteroidal anti-inflammatory medication prescribed for treatment of arthritis; or antiparkinsonian therapy for the patient who manifests extrapyramidal signs from psychotropic medication; or, as earlier, the patient who receives gout treatment for hyperuricemia resulting from thiazide therapy for essential hypertension.

I do not wish to be guilty of vigorous declamation in emphasizing MED1C. I hope that my message has been clearly imprinted in your clinical practice. In every patient encounter, take a moment to stop and ask yourself—could this medical issue be related to the patient's medicine?

Drug Interactions

We have all heard of cytochrome P450 enzymes. What is cytochrome P450 and what does it do?

Cytochrome P450 is a family of enzymes; in fact, there are more than 100 enzymes in this family. These iron-containing enzymes have a broad spectrum of biologic activity:

- Enable oxygen to be used in the cellular production of adenosine triphosphate
- Degrade exogenous substances (e.g., pollutants, chemicals)
- Degrade endogenous substances (e.g., steroids, prostaglandins)
- Metabolize medications

The nomenclature of this enzyme family is complex. The enzyme is differentiated into subfamilies and finally the specific isozyme. For example, the enzyme named CYP2E1 can be deciphered as follows:

- CYP = cytochrome P450 family of enzymes
- 2 = the subfamily of enzyme
- E = ethanol (the agent oxidized by the enzyme)
- 1 = the specific isozyme

With clinical reference to drug interactions, the enzyme CYP3A4 is most prominent in the liver hepatocytes and in the gut wall mucosal cells. This specific enzyme metabolizes the greatest number of medicines in humans.

Clinical Points About CYP3A4 Enzyme

In the liver, *concomitant ingestion* of two drugs metabolized by this enzyme will induce *competition* for the binding sites on the enzyme. This competition alters the blood levels of the medicines. The drug with the higher affinity for the enzyme is preferentially metabolized with resultant decrease in blood level. The concentration of the second drug, the one with lesser affinity for the binding sites on CYP3A4, then rises. Examples of drug competition include HMGCoA reductase inhibitors (statins) with antiretroviral HIV protease inhibitors, gemfibrozil, macrolide antibiotics, and cyclosporine.

Remember, as in this case, drug interaction may be due to competition between two drugs for the CYP3A4 enzyme.

Additionally, some drugs *impair* the activity of this enzyme. In the intestinal mucosal cells, grapefruit juice impairs the CYP3A4 enzyme. An important example of this reduced enzyme activity relates to the patient who is taking a statin medication. Concomitant intake of grapefruit juice results in increased intestinal absorption of the statin and a higher blood level of the statin, potentially increasing the risk of muscle or liver toxicity.

Remember, as in this case, an elevated drug blood level may be due to impaired CYP3A4 enzyme activity.

Certainly, not all drug interactions are related to cytochrome P450 enzymes.

Clinical vignette: A 48-year-old woman takes levothyroxine for treatment of hypothyroidism. Over a period of 2 months, she has a recurrence of her initial hypothyroid symptoms, namely, fatigue, cold intolerance, constipation, and dry skin. Concomitant with the recurrence of symptoms, the serum TSH level had increased.

Here is the key clinical point: Two months ago, treatment for osteoporosis was started, with the patient taking a biphosphonate, vitamin D, and calcium carbonate. The calcium carbonate reduces gastrointestinal absorption of levothyroxine. As a result, the patient was again hypothyroid.

In addition, other medicines containing bivalent or trivalent cations, for example, aluminum hydroxide and ferrous sulfate, reduce gastrointestinal absorption of the thyroid hormone.

Here is a final example of drug–drug interaction that can have fatal results. Patients who undergo renal allograft transplantation will take transplant medication to prevent rejection. The success of the renal allograft may be jeopardized if the patient takes St. John's wort or the anticonvulsants phenytoin and carbamazepine or the antituberculous agents isoniazid and rifampin. All of these reduce cyclosporine levels and increase the risk of acute renal rejection.

In contrast, many medicines increase cyclosporine levels. These include the calcium channel blockers verapamil, diltiazem, nicardipine, and amlodipine; the antifungals ketoconazole and fluconazole; the antibiotics erythromycin and clarithromycin; and grapefruit juice.

You must remember:
The bottom line with MED1C:
1. Whatever the patient's symptom
2. Whatever the patient's abnormal physical sign
3. Whatever the patient's abnormal laboratory value
4. Think of the patient's medication as the cause

Chapter 4

Stop . . . and Think

In the hectic pace of medical practice, it is very important for the clinician to proverbially "stop, take a breath, and think for a moment." Just stop and think. Question yourself. Is the diagnosis correct? Did I rush too quickly to judgment? Could there be something else going on with my patient?

In this chapter, I wish to illustrate the value of taking a moment to stop and think. I have attempted to identify medical topics that will hopefully pique your curiosity and, perhaps, cause you to reconsider your patient's diagnosis. Alternatively, "Stop . . . and think" may prompt you to modify therapy in a patient.

It is my intent that you will find this chapter to be interesting, informative, and valuable in patient care.

Topic 1: It May Not Be Irritable Bowel Syndrome

You have diagnosed irritable bowel syndrome (IBS) in a 34-year-old woman who has problematic abdominal bloating and loose stools. The patient is well nourished but has a persistent iron-deficiency anemia.

Stop . . . and think.

Your patient *may have celiac disease*. Of course, you are aware that celiac disease in the infant or small child causes failure to thrive, diarrhea, and malabsorption syndrome. However, in the adult, celiac disease may produce *mild gastrointestinal symptoms*; indeed, some patients may have no gastrointestinal complaints.

Celiac disease is an immunologic disease characterized by gluten intolerance and presence of antibodies to gluten, a storage protein found in wheat, rye, and barley. In all patients with celiac disease, there is malabsorption of iron, vitamin D, and calcium. Iron deficiency and osteoporosis are common secondary disorders.

Think of celiac disease in any patient who has iron deficiency anemia without evidence of gastrointestinal blood loss, deficient iron intake, or hemolytic anemia with associated hemoglobinuria.

Approximately 5% of patients who have celiac disease have dermatitis herpetiformis (DH), a pruritic papulovesicular rash that involves the extensor surface of the extremities, scalp, neck, and trunk. However, all patients with DH have the typical small bowel mucosal abnormality seen in celiac disease.

Returning to IBS for a moment: In IBS, abdominal pain is associated with *more frequent* bowel movements. In contrast, organic disease causing abdominal pain typically is associated with *fewer or no* bowel movements during the discomfort.

IBS is the most common cause of chronic diarrhea. *However, do not overlook the patient who has persistent osmotic diarrhea due to ingestion of a nonabsorbable disaccharidase, for example, sorbitol and lactulose.* Even sorbitol in chewing gum can cause loose stools.

You must remember:
1. Celiac disease in the adult mimics IBS.
2. Low-calorie sweeteners (nonabsorbable sugars) may mimic IBS.

Topic 2: Abdominal Pain May Arise in the Chest, *Not* the Abdomen

An adult patient presents in the emergency department with a chief complaint of severe right upper quadrant (RUQ) abdominal pain. Of course, you are aware this pain may arise from the biliary structures, stomach, pancreas, kidney, bowel, and the diaphragm.

Stop . . . and think.

You must remember that abdominal pain may arise in the chest; both infectious and noninfectious disorders may cause the symptom. A *non-infectious* cause of RUQ pain that originates in the chest is acute right heart failure because the elevated jugular venous pressure (JVP) is transmitted to the hepatic veins causing swelling of the liver and its capsule (Glisson capsule). Sensory fibers in the capsule cause the patient to experience pain. *In any patient presenting with abdominal pain, always assess the jugular venous pressure.*

It is common for esophagitis, acute myocardial infarction, angina pectoris, pneumothorax, and nerve entrapment to cause abdominal pain without associated chest pain. (I have seen many patients whose angina pectoris discomfort was only in the epigastrium. By the way, the location of a patient's anginal discomfort in no way indicates the anatomic location of ischemia in the heart.)

Infectious causes of RUQ pain originating in the chest include right lower lung field pneumonia or empyema, pleurodynia, viral myocarditis, and herpes zoster. The radicular pain of zoster may precede the vesicular rash by 2 to 3 days.

> Clinical vignette: A 44-year-old woman has acute right upper quadrant pain of 1 hour duration. Examination shows blood pressure of 112/76 mm Hg, pulse 104/min/regular, respiratory rate 24/min, and rectal temperature 99.2°F.
>
> Lungs are clear to auscultation, and the cardiac examination is normal. RUQ abdominal tenderness without rebound tenderness is noted. Bowel sounds are normal. There is no skin rash. The clinical impression is acute cholecystitis.
>
> Ultrasonography of the gallbladder shows normal size, normal wall thickness, and no gallstones. (This is a fairly strong indicator that the patient does not have acute cholecystitis.) Liver function tests show minimal elevation of the serum aminotransferases. Both serum bilirubin and alkaline phosphatase are normal. (This is a fairly strong indicator that the patient does not have acute hepatitis.) The chest radiograph and electrocardiography are normal.
>
> What is the diagnosis?
>
> Urgent consultation is requested. Upon inspection, the consultant immediately notes neck vein distention related to elevated JVP. The diagnosis is acute right heart failure. Ventilation perfusion scan shows multiple perfusion defects consistent with pulmonary embolism.

Assessment of JVP in this patient was essential in leading to the correct diagnosis. JVP is equal to right atrial pressure, except in superior vena cava (SVC) syndrome (discussed later). In addition to right heart failure of any etiology, you must know that there are many other conditions in which JVP assessment is essential.

Here is an important clinical point: *It is not necessary to measure the JVP in cm of water (or mm Hg). All you need to know is whether the JVP is normal or elevated.* Elevate the patient's head and chest to 45°. If the top of the venous column in the internal or external jugular vein is more than 4 cm vertically from the sternal angle, the JVP is elevated. (Yes, you can use the external jugular vein for assessment; only in the very uncommon case is the vein kinked, giving the impression of an elevated JVP. In such cases, stripping of the vein will not result in it filling from below.)

In whom should the JVP be assessed? *Here are seven clinical conditions in which JVP assessment is essential:*

- In every patient who has an *indwelling central venous line.* Central lines, for example, Portacath, may cause clotting where the SVC enters the right atrium. These patients will have an elevated JVP. (However, the right atrial pressure is normal, so the patient is not in right heart failure.) Elevation of JVP in a patient who has a central venous line without heart failure is SVC syndrome.

- In every patient who has undergone *chest radiotherapy.* Chest radiotherapy is the most common cause of constrictive pericarditis in the United States. How long does it take after the irradiation for the constriction to occur? The average is 7 years, but constriction and elevated JVP may occur as quickly as *1 month after end of radiotherapy.* You must assess JVP in every patient who has had chest radiotherapy at every visit.

- In every patient who has *chest pain.* Nearly half of patients with pulmonary embolism will have chest pain. Elevation of JVP will help in diagnosis if right heart failure exists.

    Patients with acute myocardial infarction will have elevated JVP if three complications occur:

    a. Right ventricular infarction associated with inferior wall infarction

    b. Rupture of the free ventricular wall

    c. Rupture of the ventricular septum

    Patients with acute dissection of the thoracic aorta will have chest pain, usually described as cutting or tearing. If the dissection moves proximally and ruptures into the pericardial sac, the patient will have pericardial tamponade, elevated JVP, and typically paradoxical pulse.

- In every patient who has *abdominal pain.* The preceding vignette illustrates that acute right heart failure may cause the patient to present with abdominal pain.

- In every patient who has *peripheral edema.* Peripheral edema with an *elevated* JVP suggests right heart failure (of any etiology), constrictive pericarditis, or restrictive cardiomyopathy.

    Peripheral edema with a *normal* JVP suggests medicine effect, hypothyroidism, or hypoalbuminemia related to nephrotic syndrome or liver disease.

- In every patient who has *facial edema.* Nephrotic syndrome and hypothyroidism cause facial edema, but JVP will be normal. SVC syndrome and nephritic syndrome are associated with facial edema, but JVP will be elevated.

- In every patient with *abdominal swelling*. Ascites with elevated JVP suggests constrictive pericarditis or right heart failure. (Ascites in right heart failure is usually modest.)

    Ascites with a normal JVP suggests portal hypertension, hypoalbuminemia, or intestinal or pelvic malignancy.

You must remember:
1. JVP assessment should be performed in all patients.

Topic 3: Bronchial Asthma and the Thyroid Gland

Your adult patient has long-standing bronchial asthma. Without apparent cause, the patient's dyspnea, wheezing, and breathlessness gradually worsen and are less responsive to bronchodilator and anti-inflammatory medication.

Stop . . . and think.

Adrenergic beta-2 receptors in the lung relax smooth muscle, inhibit mast cell mediator release, and increase mucociliatory transport. However, these beta-2 receptors will not express their full effect *if there is a concomitant deficiency in thyroid hormone*. In some manner, thyroid hormone sensitizes the bronchial musculature to catecholamines. Beta-2 agonist therapy will not produce its full bronchodilatory effect if thyroid hormone is deficient.

Therefore, in any asthmatic patient whose symptoms are worsening without a clearly defined cause, think of the patient also being hypothyroid; obtain thyroid function tests. If, indeed, there is even subclinical hypothyroidism, initiation of thyroid hormone replacement will improve the response of the asthmatic medication.

You must remember:
1. Thyroid hormone and endogenous catecholamines work in synergistic fashion.
2. Obtain thyroid function studies in any asthmatic patient who is not responding to therapy as expected.

Topic 4: "All That Wheezes Is Not Asthma"

Clinical vignette: An 8-year-old girl experiences wheezing and breathlessness. Auscultation of the lungs shows diffuse expiratory wheezing.

Of course, the initial impression is bronchial asthma because this condition classically includes three symptoms: wheezing, chronic dyspnea, and cough. The basic pathophysiology in bronchial asthma is airway hyperresponsiveness, for example, to methacholine.

Stop . . . and think.

Wheezing may be heard in patients who do not have asthma, but who have other conditions. Here are a few of the many nonasthmatic conditions that are associated with wheezing:

Chronic or recurrent wheezing can result from:

- Postnasal drip
- Chronic obstructive lung disease (COLD)
- Carcinoid syndrome
- Worm infestation in the lung
- Broncholithiasis

Postnasal drip is probably the most common cause of wheezing. In these patients, the expiratory musical sound is thought to arise in the vocal cords. Patients with COLD will typically manifest intermittent, bilateral wheezing dependent upon the degree of expiratory airway obstruction. Worm infestation, such as ascariasis, strongyloidiasis, and toxocariasis, is often associated with bilateral wheezing. The patients typically have other, nonpulmonary symptoms. Marked eosinophilia may be noted during the larval migration phase of the disease. The clinician must be cognizant of worm infestation in patients who have lived in endemic areas.

Eosinophilia is common in bronchial asthma, and the degree of eosinophilia appears to parallel the intensity of the disease. However, marked eosinophilia (> 2500/microL) is strongly suggestive of helminthic parasitic disease.

Carcinoid syndrome is most often related to an intestinal tumor that produces a number of various humoral agents including histamine, serotonin, and kallikreins. The classic triad of recurrent symptoms, wheezing, flushing, and diarrhea, occurs only when the intestinal tumor has metastasized to the liver.

Broncholithiasis may be most commonly due to pulmonary histoplasmosis. Calcified peribronchial lymph nodes erode into the bronchus (a "broncholith") and can be manifest by localized wheezing.

Acute wheezing can result from the following conditions:

- Acute pulmonary edema ("cardiac asthma")
- Acute pulmonary embolism
- Gastroesophageal reflux

In acute pulmonary embolism, wheezing is due to the release of bronchoconstrictive and inflammatory mediators. The wheezing is often associated with other symptoms such as dyspnea and pleuritic chest pain, and may be associated with hemoptysis. The wheezing may be localized or diffuse, dependent upon the number and location of emboli.

Diffuse wheezing may be noted in the patient who has paroxysmal nocturnal dyspnea or acute pulmonary edema. In these patients, interstitial edema causes an increase in airway obstruction that results in wheezing.

Acute wheezing in gastroesophageal reflux is common. The proposed mechanism is acidic irritation of vagal fibers in the esophagus that, in turn, activate vagal fibers innervating the bronchi. The resultant parasympathetic stimulation provokes bronchoconstriction, airway obstruction, and wheezing. Patients who have reflux often have heartburn, chest pain that may mimic angina pectoris, sore throat, water brash (hypersalivation), and hoarseness.

In summary, what are the clues that wheezing is not due to bronchial asthma?

- Sore throat
- Hemoptysis
- Postnasal drip
- Flushing
- Diarrhea
- Marked eosinophilia

Here are two important clinical topics that are related to asthma:

- Aspirin-exacerbated respiratory disease (AERD), formerly called "aspirin-induced asthma"
- Sulfite allergy

Aspirin-Exacerbated Respiratory Disease

AERD is characterized by three elements, though they do not clinically appear at the same time. Initially, the patient has chronic rhinitis, followed by development of nasal polyps and finally asthma and wheezing. The sensitivity to aspirin most commonly begins when the patient is in the third or fourth decade in age. Aspirin intake typically provokes symptoms 30 minutes to 3 hours after ingestion. Wheezing, nasal congestion, facial flushing, rhinorrhea, and periorbital edema are common symptoms.

Other nonsteroidal anti-inflammatory agents that inhibit cyclo-oxygenase 1 (COX-1) can provoke the same reaction. Interestingly, pure COX-2 inhibitors do not provoke this symptom complex.

Sulfite Allergy

You must know that there are sulfite-sensitive patients. Most, but not all, of these patients have known asthma. Ingestion of sulfites can provoke severe, even life-threatening, asthmatic attacks and angioedema.

Sulfites are used as preservatives in food and, indeed, in medications. Sulfite compounds include potassium metabisulfite, potassium bisulfite, sulfur dioxide, and sodium bisulfate. Commercial food preparations that are high in sulfite content include these:

- Dried fruit, excluding dark raisins and prunes
- Nonfrozen lemon juice
- Nonfrozen lime juice
- Wine (red and white)
- Grape juice (white, pink, and red)
- Fresh shrimp

Patients who have asthma should be counseled about sulfites, because approximately 5% of patients will experience increased wheezing and breathlessness after intake of the compounds. Sensitivity to sulfites is entirely unrelated to allergy to sulfonamide medication.

You must remember:
1. "All that wheezes is not asthma."
2. Infectious and noninfectious diseases, vascular disease, and neoplasm may be associated with wheezing.

Topic 5: Serum C-Reactive Protein and Proteinuria

Serum C-reactive protein (CRP) and proteinuria are *markers* or predictors of disease. CRP is produced in the liver and in the smooth muscle cells of an atherosclerotic plaque.

An elevated serum CRP is a predictor of the development and progression of atherosclerosis, of future coronary events including unstable angina pectoris and acute myocardial infarction, and recurrent ischemic events after both coronary bypass grafting and percutaneous coronary intervention. Serum CRP is considered to be a stronger predictor of cardiovascular events than is low-density lipoprotein cholesterol.

The clinician should know the factors that reduce serum CRP levels and engender a reduction in the incidence of cardiovascular events. These include the following:

- Exercise
- Diet high in fiber, soy, and nuts
- Smoking cessation
- Intake of HMG-CoA reductase inhibitors ("statins")
- Intake of beta adrenergic blockers
- Intake of ezetimibe

Proteinuria is a *marker* of kidney damage. Its quantity reflects the severity of renal injury. Normally, albuminuria in the normal kidney is less than 20 mg/day. Microalbuminuria is defined as persistent levels of albumin in the urine between 30 mg and 300 mg/day. For detection of *microalbuminuria*, especially in those considered to be at high risk, such as patients with hypertension or diabetes mellitus, those older than 60 years of age, or those with stage 1–3 chronic kidney disease, the spot urine *albumin* to creatinine ratio is used because it is accurate and avoids the inconvenience of a 24-hour collection. *Incidentally, the urine dipstick becomes positive when protein excretion is greater than 300 mg/day.*

Proteinuria is now also considered a *predictor* of cardiovascular disease and cardiovascular mortality, for example, from myocardial infarction and stroke, in patients with and without diabetes mellitus and with and without hypertension. The proteinuria appears to be associated with the increased vascular permeability, endothelial dysfunction, and reduced nitric oxide production that appears to be the earliest pathophysiologic abnormalities in atherosclerosis.

Stop . . . and think.

More than markers, serum CRP and proteinuria appear to be *pathogenic*.

The mouse cannot produce CRP. However, when human genes are implanted in the mouse, the *transgenic* mouse can produce CRP. Spontaneous arterial thrombosis then is noted. The CRP itself appears to be *prothrombotic*.

Experimental animal models and recent human studies suggest that albuminuria itself is pathogenic, contributing to progressive kidney injury. The albuminuria may promote the vascular endothelial injury in the glomerulus that, ultimately, causes fibrosis.

You must remember:
1. CRP and albuminuria are more than *predictors* of disease; they are both *pathogenic*.

Topic 6: Bilateral Hilar Nodes

Hodgkin's disease and sarcoidosis are the classic diseases associated with the presence of bilateral hilar adenopathy on chest radiography.

The patient with Hodgkin's disease may be asymptomatic with physical examination showing the presence of enlarged lymph nodes having a rubbery consistency. Alternatively, the patient may present with systemic symptoms including fever, night sweats, and weight loss. Bilateral hilar adenopathy is a common radiographic finding in the disease. (Non-Hodgkin's lymphoma [NHL] does not cause bilateral hilar adenopathy. However, unlike Hodgkin's disease, obstruction of the SVC is common in the patient who has NHL.)

The patient with sarcoidosis often presents with varied symptoms that may include dry cough, pain and redness in the eye due to uveitis, skin lesions, fever, malaise, and weight loss. The initial radiographic abnormality in sarcoidosis is bilateral hilar adenopathy. As the pulmonary disease progresses, the hilar nodes shrink in size with the development of diffuse reticular opacities or bilateral diffuse nodularity. Restrictive pulmonary impairment is common and may lead ultimately to severe pulmonary hypertension and cor pulmonale.

Stop . . . and think.

You must know that many other diseases may produce hilar adenopathy. Do not hasten to a diagnosis of Hodgkin's disease or sarcoidosis without considering the following disorders:

- Infectious mononucleosis
- Measles
- Pertussis

- Histoplasmosis
- Blastomycosis
- Coccidiodomycosis
- Silicosis
- Cystic fibrosis

You must remember:
1. Do not leap to a diagnosis of sarcoidosis or Hodgkin's disease in a patient who has bilateral hilar adenopathy.

Topic 7: Syncope with Effort in the Young Patient

Syncope (fainting) is a very common event in children with up to 15% experiencing a syncopal episode by the end of adolescence. Cerebral ischemia is the common denominator in all patients who faint; the etiology of the decreased brain perfusion may be benign or life-threatening.

By far the most common benign cause of syncope in the young patient is heightened vagal tone (the common faint) with its prodrome of lightheadedness, dizziness, dimmed vision, nausea, pallor, and sweating. Breath-holding syncope, typically in children 6 months to 6 years of age, is characterized by cyanotic or pallid spells. This is felt to be a variant of vasovagal syncope.

Orthostatic hypotension can cause syncope with assumption of the upright posture if the patient is hypovolemic, for example, from hemorrhage or dehydration, or is taking medication that can cause this adverse hemodynamic response.

Stop . . . and think.

The history is the most critical element in the evaluation of the patient who has a syncopal episode. The clinician must pay special heed to the young patient who faints during exertion, because this may be related to a life-threatening condition.

The clinician must think of the following conditions that can cause syncope with effort:

A. No structural heart disease
- Long QT interval syndrome
- Preexcitation syndrome

B. Structural heart disease
- Hypertrophic obstructive cardiomyopathy (HOCM)
- Anomalous coronary artery
- Arrhythmogenic right ventricular dysplasia
- Myocarditis

Long QT Syndrome

Long QT interval syndrome is an inherited genetic disorder (autosomal dominant or recessive inheritance) in which the structurally normal heart has a mutation of an ionic channel gene. As a result, abnormal myocardial cell action potentials predispose the young patient to a form of ventricular tachycardia called torsade de pointes. The arryhythmia can cause syncope, seizures, or sudden cardiac death.

You must remember three clinical facts:

- Syncope of any etiology can cause jerking of the extremities. Many children with long QT interval syndrome who faint and are observed to have jerking motion of the extremities during the episode are mistakenly diagnosed as having epilepsy.
- Long QT interval syndrome often catapults the patient into ventricular tachycardia *when the sympathetic nervous system is activated* (an adrenergic surge). Consequently, these children faint during physical effort or with adrenergic stimulation during a heated argument.
- When asymptomatic, the young patient with long QT interval syndrome will have a normal cardiac examination.

Preexcitation Syndrome

Preexcitation syndrome is a congenital disorder in which the heart appears to be structurally normal. Microscopic accessory fibers are present between atria and ventricles; these fibers enable cardiac electrical current to pass from the atria to ventricles without the normal delay in the atrioventricular (AV) node. Typically, there is intermittent conduction through these accessory fibers. When the patient is in sinus rhythm, the electrocardiographic manifestation of conduction through accessory pathways is a short PR interval, slurred upstroke of the initial portion of the QRS complex (delta wave), and prolongation of the QRS complex. At other times, when conduction of action potentials moves normally from atria through the AV node into ventricles, the electrocardiographic pattern is entirely normal.

When the ventricles are activated by current passing through these accessory fibers, the patient is at risk of fainting related to the onset of paroxysmal atrial fibrillation with a very high ventricular rate, even approaching 300 beats per minute. If the *atrial* fibrillation degenerates into *ventricular* fibrillation, sudden cardiac death results.

> Clinical vignette: A 13-year-old girl was engaged in a vigorous cheerleading routine during half-time of a middle school basketball game. She suddenly collapsed, losing consciousness. The patient spontaneously regained consciousness and was taken to the emergency department.
>
> At the time of my examination the patient was alert and asymptomatic. I carefully questioned her frightened parents because the events immediately preceding the event were of seminal importance. I was told two important facts, namely, the faint occurred during the vigorous cheerleading routine and, second, the basketball coach found the pulse to be nearly 300/min during the syncopal period. (I placed great credence on the fact that it was the coach who took the pulse, for coaches have significant medical training in their college curriculum.)
>
> My examination showed normal vital signs. The cardiopulmonary and neurologic examinations were normal. The patient's electrocardiogram was perfectly *normal.*
>
> I was impressed with two points: the faint during physical effort and the pulse rate assessed by the coach. With a perfectly normal cardiac examination and electrocardiogram, HOCM was highly unlikely. I strongly suspected preexcitation syndrome, but could not yet prove the diagnosis to be correct.
>
> I then connected the patient to the electrocardiograph machine, and while it was running, I pressed on the girl's left carotid sinus. Within 2 or 3 seconds, the electrocardiographic pattern changed from normal to the classic short PR interval and delta wave. My left carotid sinus pressure had slowed AV conduction that, in turn, caused electrical current to move from atria through the accessory fibers to the ventricles. I had proved the diagnosis of preexcitation syndrome.
>
> Subsequent electrophysiologic studies demonstrated the location of the accessory tracts. Radiofrequency ablation was successfully performed, and the patient has not experienced syncopal incidents over a long period of follow-up observation.

Hypertrophic Obstructive Cardiomyopathy

Patients with HOCM have a classic triad of symptoms, namely, exertional dyspnea (diastolic heart failure), angina pectoris, and syncope. Syncope or near-syncope typically occurs during or immediately after physical exertion.

Several pathophysiologic mechanisms may provoke cerebral ischemia and fainting. These include the following:

- Ventricular tachycardia that is related to myocardial ischemia or to fibrosis in the ventricles
- Dynamic left ventricular outflow obstruction due to apposition of the anterior mitral valve leaflet against the ventricular septum during ventricular ejection
- Hypotension related to inappropriate peripheral vasodilatation of nonexercising muscles

Arrhythmogenic Right Ventricular Dysplasia

Although common in northern Italy, particularly in young athletes, arrhythmogenic right ventricular dysplasia is rarely diagnosed in the United States. It is thought to be underrecognized in the United States. This inherited disorder is characterized by right ventricular dilation and thinning in conjunction with fatty infiltration in the right ventricle. Ventricular arrhythmias are common and cause palpitations, syncope, and sudden cardiac death.

Anomalous Coronary Artery

An anomalous coronary artery, for example, a coronary artery arising from the pulmonary artery (not from the aorta), may cause exertionally induced syncope in a child or adolescent due to ischemia-induced ventricular tachycardia. An anomalous coronary artery may cause angina pectoris in a child. If angina is to occur, it seems to begin at approximately 8 to 10 years of age. Similarly, acute myocarditis, often related to a viral infection, is associated with ventricular arrhythmia.

What I Am *Not* Saying

Indeed, it is clinically important to think of heart disorders, of both structurally normal and structurally abnormal hearts, in the child or adolescent who faints during physical effort. The syncope during effort may be related to lethal conditions. Although these conditions most likely cause syncope during physical effort, I am *not* declaring that these conditions cause syncope *only* during effort. Although thought to occur infrequently, patients with HOCM, preexcitation, and right ventricular dysplasia may faint at rest or during very light physical activity.

What You Might Not Know About Vasovagal Syncope

It is clearly recognized that vasovagal syncope is most commonly precipitated by emotional stress; noxious or painful stimuli; prolonged, motionless standing; and fear of injury. What is not well known is that vasovagal syncope is a common cause of fainting in healthy young persons during or immediately following exercise. The diagnosis of vasovagal faint has been established based upon history and tilt table testing. Exercise-related vasovagal syncope may occur in the untrained and trained athlete; may occur in those who do not have vasovagal syncope unrelated to exercise; and is associated with the same prodromal symptoms as in the patient with non-exercise-related vasovagal faint.

You must remember:
1. When encountering a young patient who has fainted during effort, consider cardiac disorders that are not associated with structural disorders as well as cardiac disorders associated with structural abnormality.

Topic 8: Is It Serious?

I suspect that the following medical conditions will be rather commonly seen in your practice. They may be entirely benign—or serious. I hope the following vignettes will cause you to *stop . . . and think.*

Urticaria: Is It Serious?

Clinical vignette: A 34-year-old woman has a 1-day history of generalized, intensely pruritic hives. The patient has no history of allergy. Two days earlier, she completed a course of a sulfa-containing medication as therapy for a urinary tract infection.

There are many causes of acute urticaria, or hives. These include IgE-mediated reactions related to foods and additives, insect stings, medications, and latex. Medicines may also provoke urticaria by direct mast cell activation, while viral and bacterial infections may cause urticaria via a complement-mediated reaction.

Could the patient's urticaria indicate a more serious condition?

You must *stop . . . and think* because there are systemic diseases that can cause urticaria. The systemic illnesses most commonly associated with hives are autoimmune thyroid disease (Hashimoto's thyroiditis and Graves' disease), systemic lupus erythematosus (SLE), Sjogren syndrome, and cryoglobulinemia.

Here are the clues that suggest urticaria is related to an underlying systemic condition:

- Fever, arthritis
- Recent arthralgia, weight loss, or bone pain
- Urticarial lesions that are *painful*
- Urticarial lesions that last more than 36 hours
- Hyperpigmentation that persists after disappearance of the urticaria

Although painful hives often are associated with systemic disease, I must point out that there are two conditions that cause painful hives *in the absence of systemic disease*. They are the following:

- Cold urticaria
- Pressure urticaria

Cold urticaria is often familial in character and is a hypersensitivity to cold. The hives may be limited to the skin areas exposed to cold or may be generalized. The skin lesions are typically burning rather than pruritic and appear approximately 30 minutes after the cold exposure, particularly during rewarming.

Pressure urticaria usually involves the hands and soles of the feet. Prolonged walking or carrying heavy bundles may provoke hives that are burning and painful rather than pruritic.

Livedo Reticularis: Is It Serious?

Clinical vignette: A healthy 34-year-old woman in a cool examining room awaits the arrival of her physician. Upon examination, the legs and lower abdomen show a fishnet, lacy purple discoloration. Livedo reticularis (LR) is diagnosed.

LR may be entirely benign in the young, healthy woman, who is usually between the ages of 20 and 40 years. It is intensified by cold and relieved by warming.

Could LR represent a more serious underlying condition?

Stop . . . and think.

LR may be an expression of an underlying systemic disease. LR is associated with the following conditions:

- Antiphospholipid syndrome (APS), which is characterized by a hypercoagulable state predisposing to recurrent deep vein thrombosis, arterial thrombosis, and recurrent fetal loss after the first trimester
- APS may be primary or related to SLE.
- In other words, LR may be associated with APS alone or may be associated with systemic lupus and APS.

Acanthosis Nigricans: Is It Serious?

Acanthosis nigricans (AN) lesions are gray-brown to black, are rough, and have prominent skin lines. They are most frequently noted in the axillae, neck, and inguinal creases. AN is associated with insulin resistance. Therefore, AN is present in patients who have diabetes mellitus, obesity, and Cushing's syndrome.

Could AN have a totally different clinical significance?

Stop . . . and think.

AN is also associated with certain cancers, most commonly, gastric and hepatocellular malignancy and, less frequently, with lung cancer or lymphoma. In the patient with AN, consider occult malignancy when the following features of AN are present:

- Rapidly progressive skin lesions
- Involvement of the mouth
- Involvement of palms and soles

Dizziness: Is It Serious?

Clinical vignette: A 41-year-old woman has a 7-day history of vertigo with each episode lasting less than 1 minute. The vertigo is described as a sense of motion and occurs when she is standing and looking up and also when rolling over in bed. At times, the vertigo is intense and is associated with nausea and vomiting.

Vital signs are normal. With the patient seated and with her neck extended and turned to one side, she is then rapidly placed in the supine position (Dix–Hallpike maneuver). The patient then experiences vertigo, and nystagmus, lasting 20 seconds, is noted.

Does nystagmus signify a potentially serious condition? Does nausea and vomiting make you think that the patient has a serious disorder? *Stop . . . and think.*

First, when a patient has dizziness, you must clearly determine what the patient is trying to tell you. *Dizziness* is a nonspecific term and may refer to vertigo, which is a sense of motion. In contrast, some patients will use the term *dizziness* to mean a feeling of presyncope or of unsteadiness (disequilibrium).

Second, you must know that vertigo may relate to *peripheral* or *central* vestibular dysfunction.

Peripheral refers to the inner ear; benign positional vertigo and Meniere's disease are peripheral causes of vertigo. Peripheral vertigo may be associated with nausea, vomiting, tinnitus, and hearing loss. However, these patients do *not* have other neurologic symptoms. Examination may show nystagmus.

Central refers to the cerebellum and brainstem. Conditions that cause central vertigo include infarction or tumor of the cerebellum or brain stem, or vertebrobasilar artery insufficiency. Patients with central vertigo always have other neurologic symptoms, often including diplopia, ataxia, visual loss, weakness, numbness, and slurred speech, in addition to nausea and vomiting. Examination may show ataxia, nystagmus, abnormal reflexes, and dysmetria, for example, abnormal finger to nose testing.

Note that in *both peripheral and central vertigo* the patient may experience nausea and vomiting and examination may show nystagmus.

Disequilibrium means imbalance in walking. It is not associated with lightheadedness, sense of motion, or impending faint. The imbalance is most commonly related to peripheral neuropathy, musculoskeletal disorders, and cervical spondylosis. Cervical spondylosis is a degenerative disc condition in the neck with associated bony growths involving the vertebral column. Compression of nerve roots or the spinal cord (myelopathy) may result. Patients commonly have radicular pain or sensory disturbances in the arms, occipital headaches, and neck pain. Imbalance with walking or urinary or bladder incontinence suggests spinal cord involvement.

You must remember:
1. Vertigo, nausea and vomiting, and nystagmus may occur in both central and peripheral vestibular dysfunction.
2. Patients who have vertigo of central origin always have other associated neurologic symptoms and signs.

Flushing: Is It Serious?

Clinical vignette, Patient A: A 50-year-old woman who has not had a menstrual period in 3 months now has recurrent episodes of flushing and sweating that last approximately 3 or 4 minutes. They are most frequent at night. Physical examination performed when the patient is asymptomatic is normal.

Clinical vignette, Patient B: A 46-year-old man has a 3-week history of paroxysmal headache, sweating, palpitations, and flushing. Examination during symptoms shows blood pressure 230/140 mm Hg, pulse 122/min/regular, and respirations 22/min. The patient's skin is moist; the scalp is particularly wet.

Stop . . . and think.

Could flushing be serious?

Flushing may be entirely benign, as in the woman who is experiencing menopausal symptoms related to decline in estrogen, in the patient who has rosacea, or in the patient who has ingested alcohol. Further, flushing is a very common adverse effect of many medications. Medicines that provoke flushing include these:

- Nicotinic acid and niacin (flushing may be prevented by having the patient ingest an aspirin before a meal and then having the patient take the niacin after that meal while swallowing a cold drink)
- Calcium channel blocker medications
- Phosphodiesterase inhibitors
- Tamoxifen

There are a number of conditions in which release of vasoactive hormones will cause flushing. Patients who have pheochromocytoma often have paroxysmal headache and sweating. Initially, the face is pallid due to tumor secretion of norepinephrine. The pallor is followed by flushing.

Medullary carcinoma of the thyroid is usually related to a solitary thyroid nodule whose hormone secretion may cause flushing and diarrhea. Renal cell carcinoma, whose classic presentation is flank pain, renal mass, and hematuria (microscopic or gross hematuria, without red cell casts) is occasionally associated with a paraneoplastic syndrome in which vasoactive substances provoke flushing.

An important clinical point: An adult male who develops a *left-sided* varicocele that does not empty with recumbency is likely to have a left renal cell carcinoma. The explanation is that the left gonadal vein drains into the left renal vein; a left renal carcinoma invading the left renal vein then will cause obstruction to gonadal vein emptying. On the right side, the anatomy is different; the right gonadal vein empties directly into the inferior vena cava.

Finally, the rare conditions systemic mastocytosis and solid mast cell tumors release histamine and prostaglandins that cause flushing and diarrhea.

You must remember:
1. Flushing may be benign and physiologic, due to medicines, or due to serious underlying disease.
2. In the patient who has flushing, begin a careful search for organic disease after the benign causes have been eliminated.

Topic 9: Aortic Valve Stenosis and Hypertrophic Obstructive Cardiomyopathy

Patients with aortic valve stenosis and HOCM share common symptoms, namely, dyspnea, angina pectoris, and syncope.

In both, the dyspnea is a manifestation of diastolic heart failure. Left ventricle (LV) hypertrophy is present in both conditions; the hypertrophic LV is noncompliant, causing elevation of mean left atrial pressure that, in turn, is transmitted back into the pulmonary capillary bed, causing interstitial lung edema and the patient's symptom of breathlessness.

Angina pectoris is, again, due to the LV hypertrophy that increases myocardial oxygen demand. The anginal discomfort may occur even in the absence of coronary atherosclerotic disease.

Syncope in severe aortic valve stenosis occurs with effort; in HOCM the syncope typically occurs during exertion or immediately afterward.

These are the common factors in the two cardiac conditions. What are the differences?

Stop . . . and think.

- HOCM is an inherited condition (autosomal dominant); aortic valve stenosis is not genetically transmitted.

- In aortic valve stenosis, the valvular obstruction leads to compensatory LV hypertrophy (obstruction → hypertrophy).
- In HOCM, the genetically induced LV hypertrophy causes the obstruction to outflow blood from LV to aorta (hypertrophy → obstruction).
- HOCM most commonly expresses itself in childhood or young adulthood.
- In aortic valve stenosis, patients born with a bicuspid aortic valve generally become symptomatic at approximately 50 years; those whose valve stenosis is due to degeneration of a tricuspid valve tend to become symptomatic at an older age, often about 80 years.

Topic 10: Bile Salts and Bile Pigments

I have long observed that students confuse bile salts and bile pigments. Although both are constituents of bile, are they of common origin? Do they have the same biologic function?

Stop . . . and think.

Bile salts are synthesized in the liver. Cholesterol is the precursor of bile salts (and steroid hormones). Based upon their chemical structure, they are considered primary or secondary. The bile salts are stored in the gallbladder and are secreted into the intestine after a meal. In the small bowel, they emulsify fats, thus enabling pancreatic lipase to continue the digestive process.

Bile salts are extensively reabsorbed (95%) in the terminal ileum. The salts are returned via the portal vein to the liver where they are again secreted into the bile for another digestive cycle. Only 5% of bile salts secreted into the bowel is lost in the feces.

Disease involving the terminal ileum, for example, Crohn's disease, or resection of the terminal ileum greatly reduces the reabsorption of bile salts for transfer back to the liver. The liver cannot compensate by significantly increasing production of bile salts. As a result, there is a deficiency of secreted bile salts in the intestine. Fat malabsorption then ensues. Further, the bile salt malabsorption leads to development of gallstones that is common in Crohn's disease.

The bile pigments bilirubin and biliverdin are degradation products of heme that was present in hemoglobin. At the end of their life span, approximately 120 days, red blood cells are phagocytosed by the reticuloendothelial system. The heme is then degraded to biliverdin continuing to formation of bilirubin. The bilirubin is conjugated with glucuronic acid in the liver to form "direct" bilirubin that is finally excreted into the bile. Bacteria in the bowel convert bilirubin to urobilinogen. Some is reabsorbed into the blood and excreted in the urine. Most of the urobilinogen undergoes further degradation and is excreted in the feces.

Why do patients with severe or chronic hemolytic anemia form gallstones? With hemolysis, large quantities of bilirubin are presented to the liver. The liver is unable to conjugate all the bilirubin to the water-soluble direct component. As a result, a greater proportion of bilirubin entering the biliary tract is the the less soluble "indirect" form. In the gallbladder the less soluble indirect bilirubin precipitates as gallstones.

See Table 4–1 for a summary of this information.

A few more clinical points about serum bilirubin levels:

- Extravascular hemolysis (destruction of erythrocytes in the spleen, bone marrow, and liver) results in increased serum indirect bilirubin values.
- Intravascular hemolysis results in increased serum indirect bilirubin values.
- Gilbert's syndrome is an inherited liver disease in which there is impairment of conjugation of bilirubin; therefore, elevation of indirect serum bilirubin results. This is a benign condition; no treatment is indicated.
- Patients who have intrahepatic cholestasis, bile duct obstruction, and metastatic tumor in the liver have increased serum direct bilirubin levels because the liver cells are able to conjugate the bilirubin but cannot normally remove it in the biliary system.
- Patients who have either elevated serum levels of indirect or direct bilirubin will develop jaundice.

Table 4–1 **Bile**

Bile Salts	Bile Pigments
Synthesized from cholesterol	Breakdown products of hemoglobin (Hgb)
Primary and secondary, from cholic acid	Hgb cleaved into globin and heme
95% reabsorbed in small bowel	Heme → biliverdin → bilirubin
Deficiency of bile or terminal ileum small disease → malabsorption	Conjugated bilirubin excreted via bile into intestine; some is reabsorbed as urobilinogen into the portal vein blood

- Dubin–Johnson syndrome is an inherited disorder in which there is elevation of the direct bilirubin fraction. These patients have normal values of other liver function tests, such as aminotransferases, alkaline phosphatase, and prothrombin time. This is a benign condition; no treatment is indicated.

Topic 11: Macrocytosis and Megaloblastosis

The patient has macrocytes, or enlarged erythrocytes, on peripheral blood smear examination. Does this mean that the bone marrow contains megaloblasts?

Stop . . . and think.

Vitamin B_{12} deficiency anemia and folate deficiency anemia are *megaloblastic* anemias. The *bone marrow* will show megaloblasts that result from impaired DNA synthesis in red blood cell precursors. The *peripheral blood* will show macrocytes and hypersegmented neutrophiles ("polys"). (I have always regarded *hypersegmented* to mean six or more lobes in the neutrophile.)

However, there are many conditions in which the peripheral blood shows macrocytes but the marrow is normal, without megaloblasts.

The following is a list of conditions that are associated with macrocytosis, but *not* with megaloblastosis. The macrocytic red blood cells may be noted upon peripheral smear examination *even without the patient having anemia*:

- Hypothyroidism
- Alcohol ingestion, even without folate deficiency
- Liver disease
- Myelodysplastic blood disorder (malignant stem cell disorder)
- Medicines (sunitinib, imatinib, hydroxurea, methotrexate, azathioprine, zidovudine)

You must remember:
1. Macrocytosis in the peripheral blood does not necessarily mean that the bone marrow has megaloblastosis.

Topic 12: Neurologic Symptoms

Numbness, tingling, weakness, dizziness, blurred or dimmed vision—all are common neurologic symptoms. Is the patient suffering from a transient ischemic attack (TIA), or migraine, or a seizure? In evaluation of neurologic symptoms, is there a clinical principle that guides the clinician to a quick and accurate diagnosis?

Stop . . . and think.

The principle that I have found to be most helpful is to divide neurologic symptoms into *positive* symptoms and *negative* symptoms. A positive symptom means that the nerve is *irritated, that the nerve is actively discharging*. The nerve may be a sensory nerve, a motor nerve, or an autonomic nerve. Irritation of a sensory nerve may provoke tingling, burning, or visual hallucinations, such as bright lights or zig-zag shapes. Positive sensory symptoms are associated with normal sensation upon examination.

Irritation of a motor nerve may cause jerking or repetitive rhythmic movements. Positive autonomic symptoms include hyperhidrosis (excessive sweating) and gustatory sweating.

A negative symptom means that the nerve is *not functioning*. Negative neurologic symptoms include weakness, loss of vision or hearing, and loss of somatic sensation. The negative symptom should be associated with loss of that sense upon examination. Negative autonomic symptoms include impotence, anhidrosis (lack of sweating), and lightheadedness upon arising due to orthostatic hypotension related to sympathetic reflex dysfunction.

Table 4–2 is a summary of positive and negative neurologic symptoms and signs as they relate to nerve fiber type.

Transient Ischemic Attack

A TIA *always* presents with *negative* symptoms. Additionally, all the neurologic manifestations of brain ischemia occur at the same time. For example, if a patient has a TIA manifest by weakness and unilateral blindness, the two symptoms will occur at the same time. Negative symptoms are associated with *negative signs* upon examination, for example, sensory loss or weakness.

Table 4–2 Positive and Negative Neurologic Symptoms (Sx) and Signs as Related to Nerve Fiber Type

Nerve Fiber	Negative Sx/Signs	Positive Sx/Signs
Motor	Weakness, atrophy, fatigability, clumsiness, hypotonia	Muscle twitches, cramps
Sensory	Sensory loss, ataxia, clumsiness	Tingling, "pins and needles," "burning"
Autonomic	Orthostatic hypotension, loss of sweating, impotence	Hyperhidrosis, gustatory sweating

Seizure and Migraine

In contrast, a seizure or an attack of migraine starts with *positive* neurologic symptoms. Tingling and visual hallucinations may be noted at the onset of migraine. A seizure may begin with a positive sensory symptom, for example, a bad smell, or may begin with jerking motions. Further in these conditions, there is a *progression* in symptoms. In migraine, the patient may note flickering, zig-zag lines that start in central vision and then progress to the periphery of the visual field, or the patient may note tingling of fingers of one hand. The tingling then progressively spreads proximally to the hand, then to the arm and even to the face. Note that positive neurologic symptoms in migraine may be *followed by the onset of negative symptoms*, for example, the visual hallucinations may be followed by a visual field defect, and the paresthesias may be followed by numbness and even extremity weakness. In a seizure, the involuntary muscle jerking may start with focal activity that is followed by anatomic progression ("march") of the motor activity.

Topic 13: The Diagnosis Is Stroke

Stop . . . and think.

Could it be a mimic of stroke?

> Clinical vignette, Patient A: An 82-year-old man has the sudden onset of right-sided weakness lasting 7 hours. Blood pressure is 146/88 mm Hg, pulse is 96/min/regular. Rectal temperature is

99.6°F. Examination shows a left carotid bruit, right hemiparesis, hemisensory deficit on the right, exaggerated deep tendon reflexes in the right extremities, and an extensor Babinski response on the right.

Did this patient have a stroke?

Clinical vignette, Patient B: A 67-year-old man has the sudden onset of left-sided weakness. Blood pressure is 136/76 mm Hg, pulse is 122/min/irregularly irregular, respiratory rate is 21/min, and rectal temperature is 99.6°F. Examination shows the apical impulse in the sixth intercostal space in the anterior axillary line, a 2/6 apical holosystolic murmur, and left hemiparesis.

Did this patient have a stroke?

Clinical vignette, Patient C: A 66-year-old woman with a long history of alcohol abuse has a 2-day history of insomnia followed by disorientation, slurred speech, and ataxia. At the time of examination, the patient is confused and agitated. Jaundice, spider telangiectasia on the shoulders, red palms, and ascites are noted. No deep tendon reflexes are elicited, but asterixis is present in both hands.

Did this patient have a stroke?

Clinical vignette, Patient D: A 34-year-old man has a 3-hour history of diffuse headache, vertigo, nausea, and vomiting. Blood pressure is 106/68 mm Hg, pulse is 118/min/regular, and respirations are 22/min. The patient is not cyanotic. Careful neurologic examination is normal. Specifically, there is no nuchal rigidity, papilledema, or nystagmus.

Note: One hour after this patient presented in the emergency department, his two sons, ages 9 and 12 years, were brought to the emergency department with similar symptoms.
Did this patient have a stroke?

Clinical vignette, Patient E: An 81-year-old man with atherosclerotic cerebrovascular disease and mild dementia is admitted to the hospital for treatment of pneumonia. While receiving supplemental oxygen and intravenous antibiotics, on the third day the patient quickly becomes confused, agitated, and at times combative. Blood pressure is 152/94 mm Hg, pulse is 112/min/regular, and respirations are 24/min. The patient is flushed, confused, agitated, and tremulous. Pupils are dilated and equal. Because of the patient's mental state, other elements of the neurologic examination could not be performed.

Did this patient have a stroke?

Here are five clinical vignettes in which patients manifest sudden or, at least, quick onset of neurologic deficit. The clinician's first thought, not unexpectedly, may be that the patient has suffered a stroke.

Stop . . . and think.

A stroke is a sudden loss of focal brain function that is most commonly the result of ischemic injury (thrombosis or embolism), but may also be related to intracerebral hemorrhage (ICH). Subarachnoid hemorrhage (SAH), typically, does not cause focal neurologic signs and symptoms.

A stroke is likely if

- There are definite focal, *negative*, neurologic symptoms
- There are definite focal, *negative*, neurologic signs
- The time of onset of symptoms can be clearly defined

The clinician must be aware that there are conditions that mimic stroke. Mimics of stroke include the following:

- Migraine
- Toxic/metabolic encephalopathy (TME)
- Seizures
- Alcohol-related disorders
- Conversion reaction
- Poisoning

TME is characterized by acute global cerebral dysfunction in the absence of structural brain disease. It often is expressed as confusion or delirium and usually is a consequence of systemic illness. Causes of TME include medicines (do you remember MED1C?), sepsis, hepatic failure, uremia, hypo- or hypernatremia, hypocalcemia, cerebral anoxia, and hypoglycemia. These patients do not exhibit *focal* neurologic symptoms or signs except rarely in the patient who has hypoglycemia or hepatic failure.

Seizures may not be associated with structural brain disease and may be inherited as in some patients with epilepsy. Acquired seizures may be due to brain tumor, intracranial infection, head trauma, degenerative brain disease, and stroke. Importantly, seizures may occur at the onset of a SAH, intracranial hemorrhage, or embolic infarction, but are *rare* at the onset of thrombotic stroke. Similarly, a seizure is not part of the clinical presentation of a TIA.

Seizures develop in 15% of *all* stroke patients. In SAH and ICH, seizures may be manifest at the onset of clinical presentation or develop for the first time weeks or months later. In contrast, thrombotic stroke may cause seizure development, but typically that starts weeks, even years, after the acute event.

Approximately 15% of migraine attacks may mimic stroke. Migraineurs may have unilateral motor or sensory symptoms lasting as long as 2 weeks. Those with basilar-type migraine have dysarthria, dizziness, vertigo, and ataxia that may suggest stroke.

Wernicke encephalopathy related to chronic alcohol abuse and thiamine deficiency is manifest as ataxia, acute confusion, and oculomotor dysfunction, often cranial nerve VI palsy, or horizontal nystagmus. The clinician may very easily consider the patient to have had a stroke.

Hypoglycemia deserves particular attention. Classically, hypoglycemic symptoms are of two types, the *autonomic* and the *neuroglycopenic*. Autonomic symptoms are due to release of norepinephrine at adrenergic postganglionic nerve endings and acetylcholine at cholinergic receptors. Symptoms include sweating, palpitations, tremulousness, hunger, and paresthesias.

Glucose deprivation in the central nervous system produces the neuroglycopenic manifestations including confusion, fatigue, seizures, and coma. Occasionally, hypoglycemia may present as focal neurologic deficit, for example, hemiplegia. The clinician must not confuse the neurologic manifestations of hypoglycemia with stroke.

An interesting note on hypoglycemic symptoms:

- Those diabetic patients with poor glycemic control tend to have autonomic symptoms during hypoglycemic periods, but
- Those diabetic patients with strict glycemic control tend to have neuroglycopenic manifestations of hypoglycemia

When was the last time that you considered poisoning as the cause of your patient's acute neurologic symptoms? The neurologic manifestations of poisons include these:

- Acutely altered mental status
- Seizures
- Peripheral neuropathy (arsenic causes the sensory, and lead the motor)

I emphasize two important clinical points that relate to poisoning: First, the acutely altered mental status will raise suspicion of stroke (as might the seizure activity) and, second, neurologic examination in the patient suffering from poisoning, in almost all cases, *will not show focal signs.*

A few causes of poisoning that can acutely change mental status include the following:

- Carbon monoxide (CO)
- Cyanide
- Gamma hydroxybutyrate
- Lysergic acid diethylamide
- Phencyclidine
- Toluene
- Methanol
- Ethylene glycol
- Ciguatera fish poisoning
- Shellfish poisoning

CO poisoning is considered to be the most common poisoning in the United States. Neurologic symptoms typically start with diffuse headache and then may progress to include weakness, vertigo, drowsiness, confusion, and seizures.

You must know that pulse oximetry and arterial blood gas values are not helpful in dignosing CO poisoning because these modalities cannot differentiate between the normal oxyhemoglobin and the pathologic carboxyhemoglobin in the poisoned CO patient. In addition, the partial pressure of oxygen in arterial blood (pO_2) represents dissolved oxygen in blood and does not represent oxygenated hemoglobin. Therefore, the arterial pO_2 is normal in the patient who has tissue hypoxia from CO poisoning.

To go further on the neurologic complications of poisoning, here is a partial list of agents that can cause seizures:

- Tabun and sarin (organophosphates)
- Carbon monoxide
- Strychnine
- Chlorinated insecticides, such as lindane, DDT
- Cyanide
- Lead
- Mercury
- Methanol
- Scorpion stings
- Petroleum distillates and solvents

To review, *stop . . . and think* when a patient presents with acute neurologic symptoms and signs. It may not be a stroke.

To emphasize the importance of poisoning, I suggest that the clinician specifically consider poisoning, particularly in a previously healthy person who presents with an acute change in mental status or with seizure activity.

Topic 14: Circumoral Paresthesias

Clinical vignette, Patient A: A 73-year-old man has dizziness, vertigo, blurred vision in both eyes, weakness and numbness on the left side, and circumoral paresthesias. During symptoms, neurologic examination shows horizontal nystagmus in addition to weakness and decreased sensation on the left side.

Clinical vignette, Patient B: A 66-year-old woman has a 1 month history of recurrent tingling, "pins and needles," sensation in her fingers, toes, and around her lips. In addition, she has recurrent muscle cramps in her fingers and palms. Vital signs are normal. Neurologic examination shows generalized hyperreflexia, normal strength, and normal sensation. Carpopedal spasm is induced by inflation of a blood pressure cuff 20 mm Hg greater than systolic blood pressure for 3 minutes (Trousseau's sign).

Clinical vignette, Patient C: A 34-year-old woman is transported to the emergency department during a panic attack. At the time of examination she describes a "pins and needles" tingling in her fingers and around her lips. The patient is tachypneic and anxious; carpopedal spasm is noted.

Paresthesias are usually described as spontaneous tingling, "pins and needles," or prickling sensations that result from heightened excitability of sensory neural pathways. Paresthesias may be of peripheral or central nervous system origin. It is important to note that paresthesias are generally associated with a normal sensory examination.

In clinical practice, paresthesias are most commonly related to injury of dorsal roots in the vertebral column, as may occur in a herniated nucleus pulposus ("slipped disc") in which the herniation protrudes laterally between adjacent vertebral bodies and compresses one or more dorsal roots. Yet, circumoral paresthesia, notably tingling around the lips, is quite common and is of varied etiology. Therefore, the clinician must *stop . . . and think* in an effort to move efficiently to the correct diagnosis.

Patient A has vertebrobasilar artery insufficiency (VBI). Common symptoms of VBI include weakness of the extremities, in either a hemi distribution or involving all limbs, numbness or paresthesias of the extremities, vertigo, and circumoral paresthesias. In fact, circumoral paresthesias are *particularly characteristic of VBI*. Vertigo is common, but *vertigo alone* is rarely due to VBI.

Why does the patient with VBI note tingling around the lips? Sensation in the face is served by the trigeminal nerve (cranial nerve V). The sensory nucleus of the trigeminal nerve originates in the medulla of the brain, an area that receives its blood supply from the basilar artery.

Patient B has hypoparathyroidism, which is most commonly due to surgical removal of the parathyroid glands or to autoimmune disease. The paresthesias are related to the increased neuromuscular irritability induced by hypocalcemia.

Patient C has hyperventilation syndrome related to anxiety. The hyperventilation causes hypocapnia (low systemic arterial pCO_2) and respiratory alkalosis. In turn, the increased pH of the blood reduces the level of *ionized calcium* in the blood. Paresthesias are noted as a result of the low ionized fraction of calcium.

There are two more important causes of circumoral paresthesias:

- Hypoglycemia
- Mercury poisoning

As noted earlier in Topic 13, autonomic manifestations of hypoglycemia provoke sweating, diaphoresis, palpitations, and paresthesias. Mercury poisoning may occur from both inorganic and organic mercury compounds; it may occur due to ingestion or inhalation. Organic mercury toxicity attacks the central nervous system first. Manifestations include hearing loss, ataxia, intention tremor, and circumoral paresthesias.

Topic 15: Atrial Fibrillation and a *Regular* Pulse

Clinical vignette, Patient A: A 45-year-old man has a 2-hour history of palpitations. Symptoms began at a party where the patient had ingested three martini cocktails. Electrocardiography shows atrial fibrillation with a fast ventricular rate. The patient is treated with intravenous verapamil that slows the ventricular response. Three hours later rhythm has reverted to normal sinus.

Clinical vignette, Patient B: An 80-year-old man has chronic systolic heart failure and chronic atrial fibrillation. Therapy for the heart failure includes an angiotensin converting enzyme inhibitor (ACEI), loop diuretic, and beta adrenergic blocker. Digoxin therapy is added because the beta blocker does not adequately slow the ventricular response.

The patient presents in your office for routine follow-up. At this time the pulse is 50/min and *regular.*

Clinical vignette, Patient C: An 83-year-old woman has chronic systolic heart failure and chronic atrial fibrillation. Therapy for the heart failure includes an ACEI, loop diuretic, and beta adrenergic blocker. Digoxin therapy is added because the beta blocker does not adequately slow the ventricular response.

The patient presents in your office for routine follow-up. At this time the pulse is 110/min and *regular.*

Why is the pulse now regular in the three patients?

Stop . . . and think.

In patients who have *paroxysmal* atrial fibrillation, it is very common for the rhythm to convert back to normal sinus rhythm, either spontaneously or in response to therapy. Therefore, the pulse will again be regular. In the two patients with systolic heart failure and chronic atrial fibrillation, the *development of a regular pulse is clearly abnormal* and necessitates investigation. In both Patient B and Patient C, the regular pulse is a manifestation of digoxin toxicity. A regular pulse at 50/min represents digoxin toxicity with an escape junctional rhythm. A regular pulse at 110/min represents digoxin toxicity with nonparoxysmal junctional tachycardia.

You must remember that the development of a regular pulse in the patient with chronic atrial fibrillation is abnormal and is usually a manifestation of digoxin toxicity. The medication must be stopped; otherwise, a more serious rhythm disturbance will follow.

Digoxin toxicity is manifest as follows:

- Atrioventricular block (first-, second-, and third-degree)
- Ventricular ectopy (ventricular premature beats and ventricular tachycardia)
- Supraventricular ectopy (atrial premature beats and atrial tachycardia)

The common precipitating factors causing digoxin toxicity include these:

- Hypokalemia, most commonly due to diarrhea or diuretics (loop or thiazide)
- Hypomagnesemia, most commonly due to diuretics (loop or thiazide) or chronic alcohol abuse

Topic 16: Peripheral Lymphadenopathy in Adults

Clinical vignette, Patient A: A 16-year-old girl has a 1-week history of fatigue, sore throat, myalgia, and low-grade fever. Examination shows soft palatal petechiae, pharyngitis, and bilateral discrete posterior cervical and inguinal adenopathy.

Clinical vignette, Patient B: A 79-year-old man has a 7-week history of anorexia, increasing weakness, and 7-pound weight loss. Examination shows a thin, pallid man with normal vital signs. Firm left supraclavicular nodes are palpated. Cardiopulmonary examination is normal. The abdomen is scaphoid; mild epigastric tenderness without mass is noted.

Clinical vignette, Patient C: A 39-year-old man has a 1-month history of progressive weakness. Blood pressure is 92/72 mm Hg, pulse is 112/min/regular, and respirations are 21/min. Auscultation of the lungs is normal. The heart is dilated with the apical impulse in the sixth intercostal space in the anterior axillary line. A diagnosis of dilated cardiomyopathy is made. The patient is treated with furosemide, lisinopril, and atenolol.

Upon examination 1 month after the therapeutic regimen has been established, the patient is clinically improved. However, he now has generalized, nontender, discrete lymphadenopathy.

Adenopathy is noted in a large number of disorders. How, then, does the location of the adenopathy help in diagnosis?

Stop . . . and think.

Preauricular nodes enlarge with infection or tumor of the scalp, the external ear or ear canal, and the *middle of the face*, for example, conjunctivitis and parotid infection or tumor. Waldeyer's ring tumors, that is, lymphoid tumor in the tonsils, adenoids, nasopharynx, and base of the tongue, and in an endemic area, Chagas disease are common causes of preauricular adenopathy.

Isolated suprascapular adenopathy is most suggestive of malignancy. Right suprascapular adenopathy is often associated with cancer in the mediastinum, lungs, or esophagus. Left suprascapular adenopathy is associated with malignancy arising in the pancreas, stomach, gallbladder, kidneys, ovaries, prostate, or testis.

In the young patient who has fever, sore throat, and myalgia, palpable posterior cervical adenopathy is more suggestive of infectious mononucleosis than is the presence of anterior adenopathy. Additionally, posterior cervical adenopathy may be noted in head and neck malignancy and lymphoma. An important clinical point: In a patient who has pharyngitis, the presence of posterior cervical, axillary, or inguinal adenopathy differentiates infectious mononucleosis from other causes.

Anterior cervical adenopathy is noted in infections of the head and neck or with such systemic infections as cytomegalovirus, infectious mononucleosis, or toxoplasmosis. Epitrochlear adenopathy is present in infections of the hand and forearm, in addition to lymphoma, sarcoidosis, and secondary syphilis. Axillary nodes may be enlarged in patients who have cancer of the breast or infections of the arm, including cat scratch fever. Inguinal adenopathy is present in patients who have infection of the lower extremity, genital or anorectal malignancy, and the sexually transmitted diseases herpes, gonococcal urethritis, lymphogranuloma venereum, and chancroid.

Generalized lymphadenopathy occurs in the infectious diseases, for example, infectious mononucleosis or HIV. In HIV, the nontender adenopathy develops in the majority of patients during the second week of symptomatic infection. Approximately half of patients who have SLE have generalized adenopathy, occurring most frequently at the onset of disease or during acute exacerbations. Many medications can cause generalized adenopathy. The list of offending medications includes these:

- Atenolol
- Allopurinol
- Penicillin/cephalosporins
- Sulfonamides
- Phenytoin
- Carbamazepine

Topic 17: Cough in the Cardiac Patient

Clinical vignette, Patient A: A 79-year-old man has an acute anterior ST segment elevation myocardial infarction (STEMI) that is not complicated by heart failure or arrhythmia. The patient is treated with aspirin, thrombolytic agent, metoprolol, and lisinopril. One week later the patient has a chronic, nonproductive cough that is worse in the recumbent position.

What is the cause of the cough?

Stop . . . and think.

The cough could be *either* an adverse effect of the lisinopril *or* because the patient developed heart failure. It is not commonly recognized that heart failure is associated with a chronic, nonproductive cough. Clinically, it is very important to correctly determine the etiology of the cough. If it is heart failure, the clinician may wish to increase the dose of the ACEI. If the cough is due to the ACEI, then it needs to be discontinued. What is the appropriate clinical approach to this case?

If the patient, after initiation of ACEI therapy, has gained weight, has pulmonary crackles, or has a new gallop rhythm, the most likely cause of the cough is heart failure. In contrast, if the patient has lost weight and has no pulmonary crackles, gallop rhythm, or peripheral edema, the most likely etiology of the cough is an adverse reaction to the lisinopril. In this case, an angiotensin receptor blocker (ARB) should be substituted for the ACEI.

Approximately 20% of patients who take an ACEI will develop a nonproductive cough. The ACEI-induced cough generally starts within 1 week of initiation of therapy, but the onset may be delayed for up to 6 months. The medication-induced cough is not more common in the asthmatic patient. Further, the ACEI does not cause or worsen outflow air obstruction in the asthmatic.

After discontinuation of ACEI medication, the cough generally recedes in 1–2 weeks, but may take as long as 1 month. Compared to ACEIs, the ARBs are much less likely to provoke coughing.

Topic 18: Angina Pectoris, Transient Ischemic Attack, and Floaters

---

Clinical vignette, Patient A: A 71-year-old man has exertional pressure in the anterior chest while walking his dog on a chilly morning.

Clinical vignette, Patient B: A 77-year-old woman has weakness and numbness of the right arm and right leg lasting 15 minutes.

Clinical vignette, Patient C: A 51-year-old woman has "cobwebs and insects" in her left visual field. They are most noticeable when she is looking at a white background. The images move as she moves her eyes.

Clearly, the patients' diagnoses are, in order, angina pectoris, TIA, and floaters.

Stop . . . and think.

The important clinical point is to determine whether the incident is the first episode (a new symptom) or whether the episode is a recurrence or even a chronic disturbance (an old symptom).

The *very first episode* of angina pectoris represents unstable angina, which is a medical emergency for which hospitalization is indicated. The *very first episode* of a TIA is an emergent situation, because the patient is at significant risk of early stroke. The *very first episode* of floaters is often related to a vitreous hemorrhage that may indicate a retinal tear. This, too, requires urgent evaluation by an ophthalmologist.

Patients with long-standing coronary heart disease and cerebrovascular disease often have recurrent transient symptoms of arterial insufficiency, namely, angina or TIA. In the patient under therapy for the atherosclerotic condition, an attack of angina or a TIA is not an emergency as long as the anginal or TIA pattern is not increasing in frequency or increasing in duration. Similarly, many patients have floaters for years, learn to live with them, and do not suffer worsening vision from their presence.

The key clinical point is that the clinician must specifically determine whether the symptom is new or old.

Topic 19: Atrial Fibrillation: Why Is It So Hard to Control the Ventricular Rate?

Clinical vignette, Patient A: A 66-year-old woman has a 1-month history of fatigue and anorexia associated with a 4-pound weight loss. One week ago, racing heart palpitations were noted; cardiac evaluation revealed atrial fibrillation with a fast ventricular response. Despite therapy with metoprolol and verapamil, the ventricular rate at rest has remained high, between 122 and 136/min.

Clinical vignette, Patient B: A 46-year-old woman has 1 hour of shortness of breath associated with nonproductive cough for which she is hospitalized. Atrial fibrillation with a ventricular rate of 140/min is noted in the emergency department. Despite therapy with a beta adrenergic blocker and non-dihydropyridine calcium channel blocker, the ventricular rate is not controlled.

Stop . . . and think.

In my clinical experience, the two most common conditions associated with atrial fibrillation in which the ventricular rate is difficult to control with medication are hyperthyroidism and pulmonary embolism.

The most likely explanation for the persistently fast ventricular response in hyperthyroidism is the fact that thyroid hormone sensitizes tissues, in this case, the AV node, in promoting the effect of catecholamines on AV conduction.

Atrial fibrillation is common in the *older* hyperthyroid patient, especially the one with "apathetic hyperthyroidism." In contrast to the classic symptoms of increased energy, insomnia, increased appetite, and heat intolerance associated with the hyperthyroid state, patients who have apathetic hyperthyroidism have anorexia, constipation, and fatigue. Atrial fibrillation is common in these patients and anticoagulation is prescribed because of increased risk of thromboembolism. As treatment returns the patient to euthyroid status, the ventricular rate is easier to control and, in many cases, spontaneous reversion to normal sinus rhythm occurs. Atrial fibrillation occurs in less than 1% of patients who are younger than age 40 years.

All patients with hyperthyroidism have lid lag, but only patients with the autoimmune Graves' disease have exophthalmus and pretibial myxedema in conjunction with the presence of anti-thyroid-stimulating hormone antibodies in the serum.

Atrial fibrillation occurs in a minority of patients who have acute pulmonary embolism, perhaps 15%. It has been my experience that, in many of these patients, the ventricular rate has been difficult to control. Factors that appear to promote tachycardia include alveolar hypoventilation, increased alveolar dead space, and the presence of intrapulmonary right to left shunting.

Risk factors for deep vein thrombosis and pulmonary embolism are well recognized. These are clinically categorized as inherited or acquired risk factors. The inherited thrombophilias, causing a hypercoagulable state, include the following:

- Factor V Leiden mutation
- Deficiency in protein C or S
- Deficiency in antithrombin III
- Prothrombin gene mutation

Acquired risk factors include, in part, the following:

- Trauma
- Major surgery
- Immobilization
- Nephrotic syndrome
- Heart failure
- Antiphospholipid antibody syndrome
- Malignancy

I do not think that clinicians fully recognize the importance of malignant disease in causing deep vein thrombosis and pulmonary embolism. Carcinoma of the pancreas, lung, prostate, kidney, and colon appear to produce a hypercoagulable state because the tumor produces a substance that increases platelet aggregation and increases coagulation factors. Importantly, the deep vein thrombosis and pulmonary embolism may precede clinical recognition of the malignancy.

Topic 20: Age Matters in Disease Presentation

Coronary Heart Disease

Clinical vignette, Patient A: An 80-year-old man faints while sitting on the side of his bed. He spontaneously awakens and is brought to the hospital emergency department. The patient is alert and oriented, mildly breathless, but not cyanotic. Blood pressure is 140/90 mm Hg, pulse is 106/min/regular, and respirations are 20/min. The JVP is normal. A few bibasilar crackles and an apical S4 gallop are heard. Electrocardiography shows ST segment depression in the lateral leads. Chest radiography shows mild interstitial edema.

Clinical vignette, Patient B: For 1 hour, an 82-year-old woman has weakness without associated cardiorespiratory, neurologic, or gastrointestinal symptoms. Vital signs are normal. Lungs are clear to auscultation; heart size is normal and a paradoxically split S2 is heard. Electrocardiography shows new complete left bundle branch block.

Stop . . . and think.
How does age affect clinical presentation of disease?

These clinical vignettes point out that older adult patients, particularly those older than 75 years in age, often do not have the severe chest pain that is classically noted in acute myocardial infarction. Rather than experiencing chest pain, older adult patients often present with one of these symptoms:

- Syncope
- Breathlessness due to heart failure
- Undue weakness or fatigue without apparent cause

Always instruct your patient who has coronary heart disease that undue fatigue or weakness is a very important symptom and that the patient must be urgently evaluated.

Note that *women of any age* may have an atypical presentation of acute myocardial infarction and have the same symptoms as the older adult patient.

Additionally, remember that electrocardiography in the older adult patient with acute myocardial infarction often does not show the typical STEMI. Electrocardiography may show ST segment depression or *new complete left bundle branch block.*

Hyperthyroidism

As noted earlier (in Topic 19), the older patient often does not have the classic manifestations of hyperthyroidism including increased energy, heat intolerance, increased appetite, tremulousness, sweating, and weight loss. Rather, the older patient is apathetic, complaining of fatigue and constipation. *Oftentimes, the older patient with hyperthyroidism presents with atrial fibrillation. Take a moment and check for lid lag in every patient who presents with new atrial fibrillation. A serum thyroid stimulating hormone level should be determined.*

Topic 21: Pulmonary Infarction and Hepatic Infarction: Why Are Infarctions of the Lung and Liver So Uncommon?

Stop . . . and think.

Infarction of the liver and lung are uncommon because both organs have a dual blood supply. The liver receives blood and oxygen primarily from the hepatic artery. In addition, the portal vein carries absorbed nutrients from the bowel and also delivers oxygen to the liver parenchyma. Today, hepatic infarction appears to be most commonly related to invasive procedures, including ligation of the hepatic artery during laparoscopic cholecystectomy, hepatic artery thrombosis after liver transplantation, and hepatic artery chemoembolization. Sickle cell disease and toxemia of pregnancy are medical disorders that may cause infarction of the liver.

The lung receives fully oxygenated blood from the bronchial arteries derived from the descending aorta and a lesser concentration of oxygen from the pulmonary arteries. Additionally, the lung parenchyma has another source of oxygen, namely, the alveoli. Two of these three must be compromised before pulmonary infarction occurs.

Thus, in a patient who has no cardiorespiratory disease, pulmonary infarction is rare. Left heart failure increases pulmonary venous pressure that, in turn, reduces bronchial artery blood flow. In the heart failure patient, a pulmonary embolus may produce infarction for two of the three oxygen sources to the lung parenchyma.

Topic 22: Pulse Pressure: A New Look at an Old Sign

Clinical vignette, Patient A: A vigorous 82-year-old man undergoes clinical examination prior to elective cataract surgery. Apart from his visual blurring, he has no symptoms. Blood pressure is 162/76 mm Hg, pulse is 88/min/regular, and respirations are 18/min. Lungs are clear to auscultation. Heart size is normal. No murmur is heard, but a soft S4 gallop is noted at the apex.

Clinical vignette, Patient B: A 47-year-old woman has a 1-month history of insomnia and heat intolerance. For the past week she has noted exertional breathlessness and mild, bilateral ankle swelling. Blood pressure is 146/62 mm Hg, pulse is 126/min/regular, and respirations are 26/min. Lid lag is present. A diffuse goiter is palpated. Bibasilar lung crackles are heard. Heart size is indeterminate; no murmurs are heard, but an S3 gallop is noted at the apex. One plus bilateral ankle edema is present. Femoral artery pulses are bounding.

Clinical vignette, Patient C: A 42-year-old asymptomatic man with known bicuspid aortic valve has a follow-up examination. Blood pressure is 140/66 mm Hg, pulse is 100/min/regular, and respiratory rate is 17/min. Jugular venous pressure is normal. Lung fields are clear to auscultation. The apex of the heart is displaced to the left and downward. A 2/6 *left sternal border* diastolic blowing murmur is heard with an apical S3 gallop.

Three patients, all different clinically, but all sharing the same sign— increased pulse pressure. What does an increased pulse pressure mean?

Stop . . . and think.

Increased pulse pressure occurs in

- Advancing age
- Hyperthyroidism
- Aortic valve regurgitation

In the older adult patient, systolic blood pressure continues to rise as a result of decreased compliance of the aorta and large arteries. The diastolic pressure does not change or may decrease slightly. This is *isolated systolic hypertension* (ISH) in older adults. *ISH is clinically important because these patients have an increased risk of heart failure, acute myocardial infarction, stroke, and cardiovascular mortality. ISH patients should be treated.* The preferred initial therapy is usually a thiazide diuretic; a long-acting dihydropyridine calcium channel blocker may, alternatively, be prescribed.

Patients with hyperthyroidism have an increased pulse pressure as a result of increased LV stroke volume and the reduced systemic vascular resistance found in this metabolic disorder. Hyperthyroidism is one cause of high cardiac output heart failure in which the patient has dyspnea, gallop rhythm, and peripheral edema despite increased left ventricular performance. Aortic valve regurgitation has an increased pulse pressure related to the increased LV stroke volume increasing systolic pressure and the diastolic regurgitant flow into the LV decreasing diastolic pressure.

Remember these clinical points about pulse pressure:

- An increased pulse pressure is an important sign.
- In the older adult patient, it may represent isolated systolic hypertension.
- ISH should be treated in an effort to reduce cardiovascular mortality.
- Aortic valve regurgitation due to aortic cusp disease typically produces a murmur loudest along the left sternal border.
- Aortic valve regurgitation due to aortic root disease, as occurs in fusiform or dissecting aortic aneurysm, often produces a diastolic regurgitant murmur that is louder (or only heard) along the right sternal border.

- Bicuspid aortic valve not only is associated with the development of aortic valve stenosis and aortic valve regurgitation, but also with the development of aortic aneurysm that may be fusiform or dissecting.

Topic 23: Diplopia

Clinical vignette, Patient A: One day after aching pain in his right eye, a 67-year-old man with type 2 diabetes mellitus awakens with double vision. Examination shows right eyelid ptosis and lateral deviation of the affected eye. The right pupil size is normal and equal to the left pupil.

Clinical vignette, Patient B: A 52-year-old man suddenly notes double vision. Examination shows left ptosis and lateral deviation of the affected eye. The left pupil size is dilated and larger than the right pupil.

Clinical vignette, Patient C: A 77-year-old woman has a 6-month history of constant blurred vision in her right eye. She now notes double vision. Examination shows no evidence of ptosis. The pupils are equal in size, extraocular movements are normal, and a dense right cataract is present.

Three patients with diplopia. What is the etiology?

Stop . . . and think.

You must determine whether the diplopia is monocular or binocular. Does the patient have diplopia only when both eyes are open, which then disappears when one eye is closed? This is *binocular* diplopia.

Obversely, does the patient note diplopia when one eye is open? This is *monocular* diplopia.

Diplopia is double vision. True diplopia is two separate, equally bright images that are visualized as a result of misalignment of the two eyes. This is *binocular* diplopia—the double vision is present only when both eyes are open and disappears when one eye is closed. Binocular diplopia may be due to congenital strabismus or inflammatory, neoplastic, metabolic, or vascular disease that impairs the cranial nerves innervating the extraocular muscles, namely, cranial nerves III, IV, and VI.

Specific causes of *binocular* diplopia include the following:

- Congenital strabismus
- Cerebral aneurysm
- Diabetes mellitus
- Hypertension
- Dyslipidemia
- Meningitis
- Multiple sclerosis (MS)
- Head trauma, usually with skull fracture
- Migraine (usually transient, but may be permanent)

Cranial nerve III (oculomotor) palsy is a common cause of binocular diplopia. It is characterized by ptosis, lateral deviation of the affected eye, and dilated pupil. An important clinical point: Diabetes mellitus is a common cause of cranial nerve III palsy, *but in 80% of cases the pupil size on the affected side is normal.*

Myasthenia gravis (MG), an autoimmune disease characterized by the presence of serum antibodies to acetylcholine receptors, is a cause of intermittent binocular diplopia. The diplopia is due to abnormal function of one of the extraocular muscles. Remember that MG affects only *skeletal* muscles; pupil size is related to *smooth* muscle function. Therefore, in MG the pupil size is always normal on the side of abnormal eye movements. All patients who have unexplained diplopia should undergo an edrophonium (Tensilon) test to determine the presence of MG.

MS often causes binocular diplopia due to cranial nerve VI (abducens nerve) palsy; this is in addition to the inflammatory optic neuritis in MS that causes eye pain and blurred vision.

Monocular diplopia is described by the patient as double vision. More specifically, it is vision with a split shadow or ghost image. The visual disturbance is present with the fellow eye covered and is not due to systemic disease, but is due to cataract, corneal abrasion, or refractive error.

Stop . . . and think.

When your patient complains of double vision, determine quickly whether it is binocular or monocular in character.

Topic 24: Neuropathies of Pregnancy

Clinical vignette, Patient A: A 32-year-old woman in the second trimester of pregnancy has burning and tingling in the thumb, index, and middle fingers of both hands. The symptoms are worse at night. Examination shows decreased sensation in the median nerve distribution. Tinel's sign and Phelan's sign are positive.

Clinical vignette, Patient B: A 29-year-old woman in the third trimester of pregnancy has the painless onset of drooping of the left side of her face and inability to close the eye on the affected side. Examination shows evidence of left peripheral facial nerve (cranial nerve VII) palsy.

Stop . . . and think.

It appears three neuropathies are increased in frequency during pregnancy:

- Carpal tunnel syndrome
- Bell's palsy
- Chorea

Carpal tunnel syndrome is very common during pregnancy and appears to be due to fluid retention that causes compression of the median nerve. Symptoms occur at any time, but most frequently start during the third trimester. Oftentimes, the carpal tunnel syndrome affects both hands and wrists. Symptoms and signs of the neuropathy disappear within weeks to months after delivery. However, it appears that symptoms may linger in those women who are breast feeding.

In the nonpregnant woman and in men, the presence of carpal tunnel syndrome affecting both hands and wrists should raise the suspicion of underlying systemic disease, such as diabetes mellitus, hypothyroidism, rheumatoid arthritis, amyloidosis, and acromegaly, in addition to the patient on long-term hemodialysis.

Chorea is uncontrolled, involuntary, asymmetrical jerking of hands, arms, shoulders, and legs that usually starts in the second trimester of pregnancy; the neuropathy resolves after delivery, though at variable times. The classic cause of chorea is acute rheumatic fever; other causes include hyperthyroidism and antiphospholipid antibody syndrome. Wilson's disease, a rare metabolic abnormality of copper transport, is characterized by liver function abnormalities and neurologic manifestations, including chorea, tremor, and rigidity.

There is a two- to fourfold increase in prevalence of Bell's palsy during pregnancy.

Topic 25: Bicuspid Aortic Valve and Dissection of the Aorta

Clinicians recognize the classic risk factors for dissection of the aorta, namely, chronic hypertension and Marfan syndrome. However, other risk factors include cocaine use, aortic vasculitis as may be present in rheumatoid arthritis, giant cell arteritis, and ankylosing spondylitis.

Stop . . . and think.

There is another condition that is gaining recognition as a potential risk factor for dissection, namely, bicuspid aortic valve (BV). Here are facts that you should know about BV:

- BV is common, occurring in 2% of neonates.
- BV is four times more common in males than in females.
- There is increasing evidence for familial clustering, with 9% of first-degree relatives having the anomaly in some studies.
- Commonly, the BV is functionally normal during childhood and early adult years.
- Almost all BV patients develop severe aortic valve stenosis or regurgitation between the ages of 40 and 60 years.
- BV patients may have an associated defect in the media of the aorta, specifically loss of smooth muscle cells, fragmentation of elastin, and increase in collagen. This pathology is related to the same arterial protein abnormality seen in Marfan syndrome patients.
- As a result, fusiform or dissecting aortic aneurysms may occur.
- All patients with BV should undergo echocardiography to determine the diameter of the aortic root.
- If transthoracic echocardiography does not clearly define the aortic root, cardiac magnetic resonance imaging or computerized tomography should be performed.
- The pregnant woman with BV and evidence of a dilated aortic root represents a special risk for aortic dissection. These patients require consideration for medicinal therapy, pregnancy termination, or cardiac surgery.

Topic 26: Petechiae, Purpura, and Ecchymosis

Clinical vignette, Patient A: A 32-year-old woman has a 2-week history of a rash on the ankles and feet bilaterally. For the past 2 days, she has had recurrent epistaxis in both nostrils requiring nasal packing. Examination in the emergency department showed gingival bleeding and nontender, nonpalpable petechiae in both ankles and feet. Platelet count is 35,000/microL.

Idiopathic thrombocytopenic purpura (ITP) is promptly diagnosed.

Clinical vignette, Patient B: An 18-year-old female college student who lives in a dormitory has a 10-hour history of diffuse headache and fever. She then becomes drowsy and nauseated, for which she is transported to the emergency department. Examination shows a febrile, lethargic patient with nuchal rigidity. Petechiae are noted on the soft palate; purpuric lesions are present on the trunk and lower legs.

Meningococcal meningitis is documented and antibiotic therapy is initiated. Chemoprophylaxis is given to close patient contacts.

Clinical vignette, Patient C: A 53-year-old man who takes warfarin for therapy of a mechanical heart valve has extensive "black and blue" marks on his abdomen and arms. Examination shows ecchymoses. International normalized ratio (INR) is 3.2.

Warfarin is discontinued. The INR returns to therapeutic levels and the warfarin is restarted at a lower dosage.

What are petechiae? What is purpura? What is ecchymosis? How do they differ from spider angiomata and telangiectasia?

Spider angiomata are dilated, tortuous arterioles that fill from the slightly raised, papular center. They blanch when pressure with a glass slide is applied to the center because the blood cells are within the vessel. As pressure is applied, pulsation of the central papule is noted, confirming the arteriolar origin. Spiders are most commonly found on the arms, shoulders, face, and upper trunk.

Telangiectasia literally means dilation of a dermal vessel at its end. They are common, asymptomatic, are not palpable, and they blanch upon pressure application. Telangiectasias may appear as discrete vessels or in clusters. They may be primary (inherited), or obversely, they may be secondary, related to scleroderma and CREST syndrome, ultraviolet radiation, corticosteroid skin atrophy, basal cell carcinoma, and rosacea.

Petechiae are tiny skin lesions that are flat, red or bluish and less than 3 mm in diameter. Petechiae represent red blood cells that have extravasated from capillaries. They do not blanch upon pressure application because the blood cells cannot be returned to the capillary circulation. Petechiae occur on mucous membranes, in the retina, and in the skin, usually first in dependent areas, such as feet and ankles. They tend to resolve in 3 to 5 days.

Purpura is simply confluent petechiae in a lesion greater than 3 mm in diameter. Purpura does not blanch upon pressure.

Ecchymosis is flat discoloration of the skin due to blood moving out of vessels. Ecchymoses undergo a series of color changes, from blue to green, yellow, and brown as heme pigment is broken down. Often due to trauma (bruising), they occur with any defect in hemostasis, both inherited or acquired, such as warfarin therapy.

Stop . . . and think.

All clinicians are aware that petechiae occur in patients who have marked *thrombocytopenia*, as in the patient with ITP. What many clinicians do not know is that petechiae may represent another, often serious, *vascular disorder*. The vascular disorder may be one of the following:

- Vasculitis, in which the vessel is inflamed with a lymphocytic infiltration. Henoch Schonlein purpura, SLE, polyarteritis nodosa, and rheumatoid arthritis are diseases that may be associated with vasculitis-induced petechiae or purpura.

- Infectious emboli that damage endothelial cells in small vessels in the skin. Infectious emboli occur in bacteremia from Gram-negative meningococcus and gonococcus; Gram-negative *Enterobacter*, Gram-positive *Staphylococcus*; and *Rickettsiae*.

- Damage to capillaries from immune complex deposition on the capillary wall, also related to an infectious disease. This occurs in subacute bacterial endocarditis and may occur in meningococcemia.

Note that infectious diseases have more than one mechanism to cause petechiae or purpura.

Here are two clinical clues that petechiae may be due to one of these vascular disorders:

- The purpuric lesions are raised ("palpable purpura").
- The purpuric lesions are tender.

What I Am *Not* Saying

I am not saying that all diseases characterized by petechiae are either related to thrombocytopenia or vasculitis. For example, patients with severe atherosclerotic disease may have plaque (cholesterol) embolism to the capillary bed that causes petechiae and purpura, or worse, gangrene ("blue toe syndrome").

Patients who sustain fractures of long bones or the pelvis are at risk for developing fat embolism syndrome. This is characterized by the following:

- Dyspnea and tachypnea from hypoxemia
- Confusion or seizures
- Petechiae or purpura

What I Am Saying

In a patient who presents with petechiae or purpura, you must do the following:

- Determine whether the purpura is tender
- Determine whether the purpura is raised and palpable
- Obtain a platelet count
- Search for a source of infection
- Obtain blood cultures, particularly if the patient is febrile
- Consider obtaining tests for serum antinuclear antibodies, anti-double-stranded DNA antibodies, and rheumatoid factor

Topic 27: The Patient with a Diffuse Rash: An Important Clue to Diagnosis

There are, seemingly, innumerable diseases characterized by a diffuse rash involving the torso and extremities. Clinicians in every discipline of medicine will encounter patients who have a diffuse rash. The rash may be infectious or noninfectious; the rash may be drug-induced or allergic or autoimmune in etiology; the character of the rash may be nodular or vesicular, petechial or ulcerated.

The clinician has a rather challenging task in determining the underlying cause of a diffuse rash. Starting with a careful description of the rash, what other clue may be extremely helpful in directing the clinician to a quick and correct diagnosis?

Stop . . . and think.

I suggest careful examination of the palms (and soles). There are relatively few diseases that are characterized by a generalized rash including involvement of the palms.

I shall divide diseases with palmar involvement into two categories, *infectious* and *noninfectious*.

Infectious diseases with a *generalized rash and palmar involvement* are these:

- Measles (rubeola) (petechiae)
- Atypical measles (petechiae)
- Smallpox (pustular rash; viral origin)
- Secondary syphilis (papulosquamous rash 6 to 8 weeks after chancre; be careful because the lesions contain *Treponema pallidum*)
- Endocarditis (palmar rash may be petechial; Osler's nodes are raised, red, and tender lesions on pads of fingers and toes, representing immune complex damage to capillaries; Janeway lesions are red papules and macules on palms and soles)
- Meningococcemia (petechiae; associated with meningitis)
- Gonococcemia (petechiae; associated with tenosynovitis and endocarditis)
- *Staphylococcus aureus* bacteremia (toxic shock syndrome) (erythema of palms followed by desquamation)
- Rocky Mountain spotted fever (petechiae; Rickettsial disease transmitted by tick)
- Dengue (petechiae and purpura; viral infection passed by *Aedes* mosquito)
- Ehrlichiosis (gram negative bacterium transmitted by tick)

Questionable infectious disease includes Kawasaki syndrome (red palms and feet with swelling of hands).

Noninfectious diseases with a *generalized rash and palmar involvement* are these:

- Erythema multiforme and Stevens Johnson syndrome (target lesions; 70% of cases have oral involvement)
- Hyperthyroidism (hyperpigmentation)
- Adrenal insufficiency (hyperpigmentation, particularly in skin creases)
- Arsenic poisoning (thickening of skin and scaling on palms and soles)
- Mercury poisoning (erythema and swelling of palms followed by desquamation)

The clinical point that I wish to emphasize is that examination of the palms and soles in a patient who has a diffuse rash on the trunk and extremities may be of key importance in leading the clinician more quickly to the underlying diagnosis.

Chapter 5

Always and Never

O ver many years in clinical practice, I have constructed personal, clinical precepts that have served my patients, and me, very well. These precepts have protected me from omission when I have been hurried; they have even prodded and challenged me to improve my clinical acumen.

I have coalesced some of these precepts into "Always and Never." I hope that you find them to be helpful.

Always

Always Consider the Medication

Always, always consider the patient's medication as the cause of his or her symptom or as the explanation for an abnormal sign upon examination.

This is a cardinal rule in medicine. I use the term *MED1C* to remind me of this principle. *MED1C* means "*Med*icine is the Number *1 C*onsideration" in every patient's symptom or observed physical sign.

A few examples:

- Pericarditis caused by medicines that have a hydrazide chemical radical, for example, isoniazid hydrazide and hydralazine
- Chemical hepatitis caused by erythromycin
- Fatal ventricular arrhythmia caused by an antihistamine prolonging the QT interval of the patient
- Confusion and hallucinations caused by a non-aspirin, nonsteroidal anti-inflammatory medication
- Dilated cardiomyopathy (left ventricular dilation and systolic heart failure) due to the chemotherapy agent doxorubicin

Please see Chapter 3, "MED1C and a Word on Drug Interactions," for more information.

Always Remember That Angina Pectoris Does Occur in Children

Angina pectoris must be in the differential diagnosis when evaluating a child or teenager who has exertional discomfort involving the chest, neck, or arms. Disorders that are associated with angina pectoris in the child or teenager include anomalous origin of the coronary artery, hypertrophic cardiomyopathy, Kawasaki disease, and cocaine use.

Anomalous origin of a coronary artery from the pulmonary artery may cause myocardial infarction or heart failure in the neonate. However, in the neonate born with adequate collateral coronary circulation, the patient may have no cardiac manifestations until the onset of angina pectoris, which may start, typically, at age 8 to 16 years.

Hypertrophic cardiomyopathy (HCM) is classically associated with three symptoms: dyspnea, syncope, and anginal chest discomfort. Onset of angina may begin as early as age 8 years, but may be delayed to the teen or young adult years. The angina pectoris in HCM is associated with normal coronary arteries.

Kawasaki disease is an inflammatory disorder of unknown etiology. Classic manifestations include fever, bilateral conjunctivitis, rash, arthritis, and lymphadenopathy. Complications of the disease include coronary artery aneurysm formation and arteritis that may cause angina pectoris or myocardial infarction.

Cocaine use results in increased norepinephrine effect at alpha and beta cardiovascular receptors resulting in tachycardia, hypertension, and coronary artery constriction. Angina pectoris may result from the combination of increased oxygen demand of the myocardium while the coronary arteries are in spasm. In addition to angina pectoris, cocaine use may precipitate acute myocardial infarction (AMI), supraventricular and ventricular arrhythmias, noninfectious myocarditis, and acute dissection of the aorta. Ephedrine-containing substances, for example, "herbal ecstasy," may cause similar hyperadrenergic activity.

Always Measure the Blood Pressure in Both Arms

Observation of unequal blood pressure levels can be of critical clinical importance in diagnosis.

Clinical vignette: A 77-year-old man with chronic hypertension has the sudden onset of severe tearing pain in his anterior chest. Blood pressure is 170/90 mm Hg in the left arm; right arm blood pressure is 130/90 mm Hg. What is the most likely diagnosis?

The answer, of course, is dissection of the ascending aorta.

Aortic dissection, with its initial intimal tear and hematoma formation in the media of the aorta, frequently causes obstruction of a major artery in the upper thorax. As a result, blood pressure levels may be different in the two arms, or the patient's physical examination may demonstrate loss of an arterial pulse in the neck, arm, or leg. The most common risk factor for dissection is chronic hypertension. Marfan syndrome, a heritable autosomal dominant disorder of connective tissue, is associated with both dissecting and fusiform aneurysms of the aorta. Congenital anomalies associated with dissection also include coarctation of the aorta and bicuspid aortic valve. In addition to Marfan syndrome, another disorder of connective tissue, Ehlers-Danlos syndrome, is associated with dissection. The abrupt, transient increase in blood pressure associated with crack cocaine use may provoke an intimal tear in the aorta with attendant dissection.

> Clinical vignette: An 81-year-old man has had two episodes, each lasting 3 to 8 minutes, of dizziness, bilateral blurred vision, and unstable gait. Blood pressure in the right arm, sitting, is 160/80 mm Hg and in the left arm, 122/76 mm Hg. When the patient is asymptomatic, the neurologic examination is normal. Which of the following is the most likely diagnosis?

Answer: subclavian steal syndrome.

Subclavian steal syndrome is most commonly caused by atherosclerotic narrowing of the subclavian artery and is more common on the left side. The arterial stenosis results in *retrograde flow in the ipsilateral vertebral artery* that causes vertebrobasilar artery insufficiency manifest by bilateral blurred vision, diplopia, dizziness and vertigo, and ataxia. Physical examination shows a significantly lower systolic blood pressure on the affected side, usually greater than 25 mm Hg.

Further, subclavian steal syndrome may have a different clinical presentation, namely, *arm claudication*. In the presence of subclavian artery stenosis, arm movement on the affected side may cause the patient to experience uncomfortable aching, tingling, and a feeling of numbness in the arm muscles.

Clinical question: In a patient who has a coarctation of the aorta, is the blood pressure equal in the arms? Answer: "It depends."

Most patients with coarctation have the congenital narrowing in the aorta *distal* to the origin of the left subclavian artery. In these patients, the blood pressure is elevated and is *equal* in the two arms. In the minority of coarctation patients, the narrowing is proximal to the left subclavian artery; in these patients, the blood pressure is significantly lower in the left arm. All patients with coarctation have radial-femoral pulse lag on examination.

Approximately 60% of coarctation patients have a bicuspid aortic valve and 10% have congenital intracranial aneurysm.

The clinician may note unequal blood pressure levels in the arms in a patient who has a thoracic aortic aneurysm, even one that is asymptomatic. The aneurysm may cause compression of a major artery in the upper chest, thus causing the unequal hemodynamic value. Takayasu arteritis, a rare inflammatory disease of major arteries that primarily affects women, may be associated with unequal pressure in the arms.

Always Consider Patent Foramen Ovale, Factor V Leiden Mutation, and Antiphospholipid Antibody Syndrome

In the young patient who has an acute ischemic neurologic event (transient ischemic attack or stroke), *always* think of patent foramen ovale, Factor V Leiden mutation, and antiphospholipid antibody syndrome.

Please refer to Chapter 1, "Medical Brevities."

Always Be Mindful of the Clinical Significance of the "Silent Ones": Silent Myocardial Ischemia and Silent Atrial Fibrillation

Silent myocardial ischemia (SI) is ischemia *without anginal discomfort or anginal equivalent*, that is, ischemia-induced dyspnea. SI is often diagnosed in the asymptomatic patient by the appearance of horizontal ST segment depression during ambulatory monitoring or during exercise treadmill testing. The pathophysiologic basis is most commonly an increased myocardial oxygen demand related to an increase in heart rate and blood pressure ("double product"). However, a significant number of episodes are thought related to *decreased coronary perfusion rather than to increased myocardial oxygen demand.*

The clinical features of SI are important:

- SI is the most common manifestation of coronary heart disease.
- SI is predictive of increased coronary events, that is, AMI, unstable angina pectoris, sudden cardiac death, and overall cardiac mortality.
- Most SI episodes occur at rest or during minimal physical activity.
- SI is most common between the hours of 6 a.m. and noon.
- Patients with diabetes mellitus or prior myocardial infarction are most susceptible to SI.
- SI occurs in patients who *have angina pectoris*, that is, symptomatic myocardial ischemia, and those patients who *do not have angina pectoris*.

- The preferred diagnostic modality is exercise testing with radionuclide imaging. False-positive and false-negative responses are more common in ambulatory monitoring electrocardiography.

Silent atrial fibrillation (SAF) is defined as episodes of atrial fibrillation (AF) that are unrecognized by the patient. Specifically, the patient has no palpitations, dyspnea, angina pectoris, or lightheadedness during the arrhythmia. The clinical features of SAF are important:

- In patients who have *symptomatic paroxysmal* AF, ambulatory monitoring has demonstrated that SAF occurs 10 to 12 times more frequently than symptomatic AF.
- Patients with SAF are at increased risk of developing heart failure because their arrhythmia is unrecognized and untreated.
- Patients with *rare episodes of symptomatic AF* may be having frequent episodes of SAF, thus increasing risk of systemic embolization.
- The clinician must be more likely to prescribe anticoagulants in the patient who has only *rare symptomatic episodes* of AF.

Always "Mind the Gaps"

In the London, England, Underground stations, there is a repetitive public address system announcement, "Mind the Gap." This refers to the fact that there is a vertical distance that separates the level of the subway train's floor and the level of the station platform. As I recall, there can be as much as a 4-inch "gap" between these two levels.

In medicine, I try always to mind two gaps that have significant clinical importance, the *anion gap* and the *osmolal gap*.

Anion Gap

The arterial blood gas (ABG) is essential in determining the acid content of arterial blood.

The clinician should arithmetically calculate the anion gap in every patient who has *metabolic acidosis* (MA). In practical terms, anion gap equals the serum sodium (cation) concentration minus the sum of (anions) serum bicarbonate and chloride.

$$\textbf{Anion gap} = \textbf{Na} - (\textbf{HCO3} + \textbf{Cl}).$$

The upper limit of normal in this calculation is 12. Greater than 12 represents an increased anion gap.

In a *normal anion gap* MA, the decrease in bicarbonate is replaced by increased chloride (Cl). Therefore, referring to the preceding anion gap equation, the increase in Cl keeps the anion gap in the normal range. This occurs in MA resulting from severe diarrhea or in patients with type 2 renal tubular acidosis, for in these conditions the kidneys retain chloride.

In contrast, in *increased anion gap* MA, the retained acid is not hydrochloric acid (HCl). *Increased anion gap* MA occurs in lactic acidosis, diabetic ketoacidosis, uremic acidosis, and poisoning caused by ingestion of ethylene glycol or aspirin. In diabetic ketoacidosis, the profound lack of insulin causes an increase in ketone bodies, primarily acetoacetate and beta-hydroxyburate. These are retained organic acids that cause MA. In the preceding equation for anion gap, the Cl is low and, therefore, the gap is increased.

In uremic acidosis, the retained acid is not HCl, but rather acids bound to sulfate, urates, and phosphate. Lactic acidosis is due to systemic hypoperfusion or malignancy. In lactic acidosis, Cl is not retained. Rather, lactic acid accumulates in the blood, resulting in increased anion gap MA. Similarly, in aspirin poisoning and ethylene glycol poisoning, Cl is not retained.

While on the subject of MA, I wish to remind you of an important clinical point. There are three reasons why an ABG study should be performed in a patient. Order an ABG if you suspect one of the following conditions:

- Hypoventilation with elevated $PaCO_2$
- Hypoxemia with reduced PaO_2
- Acid–base imbalance with abnormal pH

Osmolal Gap

First, a brief reminder in basic physiology: Total body water is in two major compartments, intracellular and extracellular. In turn, the extracellular compartment is divided into the intravascular space and the interstitial space (ICS). Osmolality is the factor that influences water movement across all cell membranes. It is water movement that attempts to maintain an equal osmolality in the intracellular compartment, the ICS, and within blood vessels.

In the normal person, the primary solutes are sodium, glucose, and urea. Because of its concentration in the plasma, the primary determinant of plasma osmolality, as noted in the calculated formula, is serum sodium *concentration* (not total body sodium).

$$\text{Plasma osmolality (Posm)} = (2 \times Na) + (\text{Blood glucose} / 18) + (BUN / 2.8)$$

The normal plasma osmolality is 275–293 mosm/kg H_2O.

The *osmolal gap* is the difference between the *calculated osmolality* (in the preceding equation) and the *measured osmolality in the laboratory* (using the freezing point depression method). A value in which the measured osmolality is greater than 10 mosm/kg above the calculated osmolality represents an *osmolal gap*. An osmolal gap indicates the presence of unmeasured union-ized compounds.

Osmolal gap = Laboratory measured osmolality > 10 mosm/kg over calculated osmolality

The most common clinical setting in which an osmolal gap is present is acute ethanol intoxication. In this condition, the ethanol has a significant influence upon measured osmolality. Osmolal gap is also important in defining the cause of MA because an osmolal gap occurs in toxic alcohol ingestion, for example, ingestion of ethylene glycol, methyl alcohol, or iso-propyl alcohol.

Finally, determining the presence of an osmolal gap assists in the evalua-tion of patients who have hyponatremia. The presence of an osmolal gap points to hyperlipidemia or hyperproteinemia, for example, multiple myeloma, as the etiology of the low sodium concentration.

You must remember:
1. In the patient who has MA, calculate the anion gap.
2. In the patient who has hyponatremia or in the patient suspected of toxic alcohol ingestion, determine the osmolal gap.

Always Determine Heart Rate at Rest and After Exertion

In a patient who has AF, *always* determine the heart rate *at rest and immedi-ately after modest exertion.*

It was William Congreve, not Shakespeare, who wrote, "Heaven has no rage like love to hatred turned / Nor hell a fury like a woman scorned." The fury of the scorned woman, however, may be no greater than that of a surgeon whose patient has an emergent, yet *preventable*, medical complication that arises during an operative procedure.

Clinical vignette: A vigorous 81-year-old man has disturbing fatigue. Evaluation shows anemia related to a small gastric carci-noma. The patient's internist performs preoperative clearance. This patient, who takes no medication, is found to be in AF with a resting ventricular rate in the 60 to 66/min range. The patient is cleared for the procedure. The abdomen is opened and the patient catapults into pulmonary edema. The patient is markedly hypoxemic; AF with a ventricular rate of 148/min is noted on the cardiac monitor. Emergently, the anesthesiologist administers medication that slows the heart rate and the acute pulmonary congestion begins to resolve.

Let us, proverbially, step back to determine what happened in this case. Transmission of the cardiac impulse from the atria to the ventricles through the atrioventricular (AV) node, that is, AV conduction, is dependent upon functional and anatomic features.

In the patient who has a diseased heart, delayed AV conduction causing AV block is commonly a result of *anatomic fibrosis* in the nodal tissues related to ischemic heart disease, valvular disease, or idiopathic fibrosis. In these cases of structural, anatomic abnormality, the AV block is permanent. *Functional slowing* of AV conduction, caused by medications or autonomic tone, is transient. Drugs such as digoxin, beta adrenergic blockers, the calcium channel blockers verapamil and diltiazem, and amiodarone slow AV conduction and may cause AV block.

Autonomic tone has a very important influence on AV conduction in both the normal person and the patient who has heart disease. Both parasympathetic and sympathetic fibers innervate the AV node. Vagal parasympathetic fibers release acetylcholine at nerve endings in the AV nodal tissues. As a result, vagal stimulation causes a decreased excitability of AV junctional fibers between the atrial musculature and the AV node, thereby slowing the cardiac impulse into the ventricles. Sympathetic stimulation has the opposite effect of parasympathetic stimulation and increases the rate of conduction through the AV node.

The patient in the clinical vignette had a *slow, resting ventricular rate due to heightened vagal tone at rest*. With preoperative anticholinergic medication and the emotional (adrenergic) stress of surgery, AV conduction was accelerated, causing the patient to go into pulmonary edema with a very fast ventricular rate. Clearly, the slow heart rate at rest was not due to structural, anatomic disease in the AV node, because the patient was able to manifest a fast ventricular rate causing pulmonary edema.

During the preoperative medical examination of the patient in the clinical vignette, the patient should have been instructed to walk for about 1 minute. The mild exercise would have reduced parasympathetic vagal tone. Without doubt, rechecking the heart rate would have demonstrated a significant increase in heart rate and the conclusion that the patient did, in fact, require medication to control his ventricular rate during surgery and after hospital discharge.

Remember this clinical point: In the patient who has AF and is taking medication to control the ventricular response, for example, verapamil or diltiazem, a beta adrenergic blocker, or digoxin, it is still important to measure heart rate at rest and immediately after exertion, *because the resting ventricular response represents the sum of medication effect and vagal tone.* Only by having the patient walk, with its effect of reducing vagal tone, will the clinician be able to confidently determine effective control of the heart rate in the AF patient during usual or vigorous activity.

Always Consider Secondary Hypertension

In the hypertensive patient, *always* remember the clues that suggest *secondary hypertension* and not essential hypertension.

Although uncommon, approximately 5% of hypertensive patients do not have essential hypertension and, rather, have a secondary cause. Here are clues that you must always remember:

- Resistant hypertension, or hypertension that suddenly develops or worsens, suggests renal artery stenosis, particularly in the patient who has signs of diffuse atherosclerosis.
- Worsening blood pressure or a significant decrease in renal function studies upon initiation of angiotensin converting enzyme (ACE) or angiotensin receptor blocker (ARB) therapy suggests bilateral renal artery stenosis.
- Resistant hypertension also raises the likelihood of sleep apnea as an important underlying condition. All patients with sleep apnea have snoring. (However, not all patients who snore have sleep apnea.)
- Hypokalemia suggests primary aldosteronism, but be aware that less than 50% of patients who have proven primary hyperaldosteronism have hypokalemia.
- Palpitations, headaches, and sweats suggest pheochromocytoma.
- Moon facies, depressed striae, and hyperglycemia suggest hypercortisolism, for example, Cushing's syndrome, adrenal hyperplasia, or neoplasm.
- Presence of a radial-femoral artery pulse lag suggests coarctation of the aorta.

Always Assess Jugular Venous Pressure

Always assess the jugular (central) venous pressure (JVP) in any patient who has any of the following symptoms, signs, or history:

Symptoms

- Chest pain
- Dyspnea
- Abdominal pain

Signs

- Peripheral edema
- Ascites
- Arm or facial swelling
- Suffusion of the face

History

- Chest irradiation
- Indwelling central venous catheter

Remember this important clinical point: It is not important to determine the exact value of JVP in mm Hg (or cm H_2O). *Rather, it is clinically important for the clinician to determine whether the JVP is normal or elevated.*

In the patient who has chest pain, the clinician must consider the potentially life-threatening conditions AMI, acute pericarditis, dissection of the aorta, and pulmonary embolism. Let us consider the importance of JVP assessment in patients who have acute chest pain.

Dissection of the aorta, most commonly related to chronic hypertension, Marfan syndrome, or crack cocaine use, may rupture into the pericardial sac causing pericardial tamponade and elevation of JVP. Pericardial (cardiac) tamponade may be a complication of pericarditis related to neoplasia, uremia, and, even, idiopathic pericarditis. In contrast to viral and bacterial pericarditis, neoplastic invasion of the pericardium is often *painless*.

In the patient who has an AMI, there are four complications that elevate JVP:

- Rupture of the ventricular septum
- Rupture of the ventricular free wall
- Hemorrhagic pericarditis
- Right ventricular infarction

Although distinctly uncommon, the clinician must recognize these AMI complications.

Acute pulmonary embolism is a common cause of acute chest pain. The patient may be in acute right heart failure with elevation of JVP due to acute elevation of pulmonary artery pressure. Other patients may not have acute chest pain but may have other disorders that cause right heart failure and elevation of JVP.

The most common cause of right heart failure is *chronic systolic left heart failure* that may be related to ischemic, hypertensive, or valvular disease or to dilated cardiomyopathy. Pulmonary hypertension due to pulmonary arterial obstruction, for example, acute pulmonary embolism, and to pulmonary parenchymal disease, for example, chronic bronchitis or pulmonary fibrosis, may cause right heart failure with elevated JVP. Chronic bronchitis and pulmonary fibrosis are causes of cor pulmonale, namely, heart disease secondary to lung disease.

The most common cause of constrictive pericarditis in the United States is prior chest irradiation, usually for carcinoma of the lung or breast, or lymphoma. The *average* interval between the radiotherapy and onset of constriction is 7 years. However, effusive, constrictive pericarditis may occur as quickly as *1 month after the end of radiotherapy*. In the patient who has had chest radiotherapy, the clinician should assess the JVP at every visit. The elevation of JVP may be noted before the patient has the marked signs of ascites, congestive hepatomegaly, and bilateral peripheral edema.

Superior vena cava (SVC) syndrome results from obstruction of blood flow from the SVC into the right atrium. It is characterized by facial and arm swelling, cyanosis, and elevation of JVP. SVC syndrome is related to malignancy, most commonly, small cell carcinoma of the lung or non-Hodgkin's lymphoma, or to indwelling central venous catheters. SVC syndrome does not cause edema of the lower extremities.

Always Educate Patients About Daily Weight

In the patient under treatment for heart failure, *always* instruct the patient to record his or her daily weight and to call if there is a 4-pound weight gain over a baseline, designated weight.

Peripheral edema is increased fluid in the ICS. The ICS, of course, is part of the extracellular compartment of body fluids. In the average adult, edema becomes evident when the patient has gained 6 pounds, that being equivalent to the body having accumulated nearly 3 liters of water.

Daily weight recording is the best clinical indicator of shifts in extracellular fluid volume.

Weight gain is often the first sign of recurrent heart failure. By recording daily weight and having the patient call if a 4-pound weight gain occurs, the clinician will have the ability to examine the patient before symptomatic heart failure recurs. I have often noted that the weight gain attendant to recrudescent heart failure is associated with the presence of a new gallop rhythm even in the absence of pulmonary crackles. The clinician can now modify the therapy and, oftentimes, prevent hospitalization. If, alternatively, the clinician deems that the weight gain is due to increased body fat, he or she can address that issue appropriately.

I suggest the following schema in instructing the heart failure patient:

- Set a "normal" dry weight for the patient.
- Have the patient weigh himself or herself every morning upon awakening, after urinating, but before breakfast.
- Have the patient call if a 4-pound weight gain occurs.

Note: The weight gain is not limited by a time factor. In other words, the 4-pound gain may be over 1 week, or 3 weeks, or longer.

Always Remember the Washout Period

Always remember the washout period of approximately 6 hours per day in the patient who takes a long-acting nitrate preparation.

Vascular reactivity to a nitrate is lessened when there is a continuous blood level of the medication. The veins and arterioles become tolerant to the nitrate, meaning that the vessels lose their dilation response. A washout period enables the vascular bed to again regain its responsiveness to the nitrate. Therefore, the clinician must use judgment in prescribing the nitrate. If the patient, for example, has nocturnal angina, the patient may take the long-acting nitrate at bedtime, but take no nitrate upon arising in the morning. Alternatively, if another patient has anginal discomfort during the morning or early afternoon hours, the patient should take the nitrate in the morning, but not at bedtime.

An important clinical point: There is *no tolerance to sublingual nitroglycerin*. The duration of its action is short, 20 to 30 minutes, and it is taken intermittently. Therefore, the patient need not be alarmed that the medication will be ineffective if taken too frequently.

Always Investigate Symptoms Associated with Vertigo and Dizziness

In the patient who has vertigo or dizziness, *always* specifically inquire about associated diplopia, ataxia, visual loss, slurred speech, weakness, and numbness.

Dizziness is a nonspecific term and may apply to presyncope, disequilibrium, and vertigo. Presyncope refers to "almost blacking out" from diffuse cerebral hypoperfusion that may occur with arrhythmia, orthostatic hypotension, or vasovagal reflex mechanism. Disequilibrium is an imbalance in walking. Cervical spondylosis, peripheral neuropathy, and primary muscle diseases may cause this gait instability.

Vertigo is a sensation of movement. It can be related to peripheral or central vestibular function. The peripheral system refers to the inner ear; the central refers to the brain stem and cerebellum. Peripheral vertigo is *not typically associated with other neurologic symptoms*. Benign positional vertigo and Meniere's disease represent peripheral causes of vertigo.

Central vertigo *is associated with other neurologic symptoms* that may include visual loss or diplopia, slurred speech, weakness, or numbness. Central causes of vertigo include VBI, brain stem infarction, and cerebellar infarction. During a transient ischemic attack involving the posterior brain circulation (VBI), the vertigo and associated symptoms are present only during the transient brain ischemia.

Always Consider Systemic Lupus Erythematosus

Always think first of systemic lupus erythematosus (SLE) in any woman who presents with acute pericarditis.

SLE is an autoimmune disease that commonly affects the skin, joints, nervous system, kidneys, vasculature, serosal surfaces, and heart. A malar rash ("butterfly" rash) or a rash in sun-exposed areas, polyarthritis involving small joints, and Raynaud's phenomenon are frequent presenting symptoms.

The important clinical point is that pericarditis is common and *often is the first clinical manifestation* of SLE. More women than men have SLE, and the disease is most commonly diagnosed during reproductive years. Between menarche and menopause, SLE has a female to male ratio of 9:1. In children (20% of cases present before age 16), the gender ratio of female to male is 3:1.

Thus, any woman presenting with acute pericarditis should have diagnostic antibody tests for SLE, for example, anti-nuclear, anti-Sm, anti-ds DNA antibodies. Anemia, leucopenia, and thrombocytopenia are frequently noted hematologic abnormalities.

Always Vaccinate Patients with Splenectomy or Impaired Spleen Function

In the patient who has undergone surgical splenectomy or has impaired splenic function, for example, splenic infarction in sickle cell anemia, *always* administer vaccines against the encapsulated bacteria *Streptococcus pneumoniae*, *Haemophilus influenza*, and *Neisseria meningitidis*.

The spleen is the primary site for production of immunoglobulin M antibodies that opsonize encapsulated bacteria. Thus, the patient with impaired splenic function, as a result of surgical splenectomy, autoinfarction, congenital absence, or related splenic artery thrombosis, is at risk for sepsis caused by encapsulated bacteria.

At least 2 weeks before the patient's elective splenectomy, the clinician should administer pneumococcal vaccine, *Haemophilus* B conjugate vaccine, and meningococcal vaccines.

Always Consider Metabolic Disorders

In a patient who presents with a psychiatric disturbance, *always* think of a metabolic disorder as the underlying cause.

Anxiety, fatigue, depression, emotional lability, and insomnia are common patient symptoms. Frequently, the clinician initiates therapy with a psychotropic agent for a *purely emotional disorder* without careful consideration of whether the patient may have a *metabolic disorder* that is causing the psychiatric symptoms.

Table 5–1 lists some examples of metabolic disorders and their psychiatric manifestations.

And *always* consider a patient's medication as the cause of psychiatric disturbance.

Please see Chapter 1, "Medical Brevities," for a more complete discussion of this subject.

Always Consider Hyperthyroidism and Pulmonary Embolism

In the patient with AF whose ventricular rate is difficult to control, *always* consider hyperthyroidism or pulmonary embolism.

Control of ventricular rate is one of the cardinal elements in the therapy of the patient who has AF. The clinician is well aware that there are times when there is difficulty in controlling the ventricular rate with beta adrenergic blockers, the calcium channel blockers verapamil and diltiazem, and digoxin. Clearly, ventricular rate control can be difficult in the heart failure patient because of associated tissue hypoxia and increased catecholamine levels. As the hemodynamic consequences of heart failure are lessened, the ventricular rate is easier to control.

The clinician may find it difficult to control ventricular rate in the patient with anemia and AF. Rate control is difficult because of the pathophysiologic effects of anemia, including decreased systemic vascular resistance, increased stroke volume, and increased tissue extraction of oxygen.

Consider the patient with AF who is neither anemic nor in heart failure. It is in this patient that hyperthyroidism or pulmonary embolism should be considered when the clinician encounters difficulty in ventricular rate control. The hyperthyroid state is associated with increased adrenergic tone that appears to be responsible for the persistently fast ventricular response in AF.

The ventricular rate may be difficult to control even when the patient is not in clinically apparent high cardiac output failure.

AF is common in patients who have pulmonary embolism; it occurs in approximately 15% of cases. Pulmonary embolism is associated with multiple pathophysiologic mechanisms that result in impaired gas exchange with increased alveolar dead space, alveolar hypoventilation, and intrapulmonary right to left shunting. These mechanisms appear related to the decreased ability of medication to slow the ventricular response in AF.

Always Try to Re-Create the Situation

In the patient who has puzzling symptoms, *always* try to re-create the situation in which symptoms occur.

> **Clinical vignette: A 36-year-old man complained of severe, diffuse headaches occurring only when walking. Examinations performed by an internist and a neurologist, followed by brain imaging studies, were normal.**
>
> **The patient was referred to me for consultation. At rest, while asymptomatic, blood pressure was 130/80 mm Hg with regular heart rate at 76/min. Physical examination was normal.** *I instructed the patient to walk in an effort to provoke the headache.* **Upon onset of the headache, blood pressure was 222/126 mm Hg with pulse of 114/min. Urinary catecholamine studies confirmed the diagnosis of pheochromocytoma.**

Pheochromocytomas may cause persistent or episodic hypertension. The classic clinical triad includes paroxysmal hypertension, sweating, and tachy-

Table 5–1 Metabolic Disorders and Their Psychiatric Manifestations

	Anxiety	*Depression*	*Weakness*	*Fatigue*	*Irritability*
Hypercalcemia		X	X	X	
Hypocalcemia	X	X			
Adrenal insufficiency		X	X	X	
Hyperthyroidism	X		X		X
Hypercortisolism	X	X			
Hypothyroidism		X			
Pheochromocytoma	X				
Intermittent porphyria	X	X			X

cardia. However, oftentimes, the patient presents in an atypical fashion, as in this case. Physical exertion, albeit mild, was associated with the sympathetic tumor releasing norepinephrine, causing onset of headache.

Clinical vignette: A 77-year-old man presented to his physician with a complaint of lower sternal "indigestion" that occurred regularly 10–15 minutes after finishing a large meal. The patient had no discomfort with physical exertion and there were no other specific cardiorespiratory symptoms. Physical examination and electrocardiography while the patient was asymptomatic were normal. Therapeutic regimens, including antacids, a proton pump inhibitor, and a histamine type 2 receptor antagonist, did not prevent the discomfort.

The patient was referred to me for consultation. At the time of my initial examination, he was asymptomatic; examination was unremarkable. Resting electrocardiogram was normal. I instructed the patient to return to my office in a fasting state, but to bring a full meal with him. At the time of reexamination in the fasting state, the vital signs were normal. Cardiopulmonary examination, followed by electrocardiography, were normal.

The patient then ate his meal in the examination room. Ten minutes after finishing, he experienced the sternal discomfort. The patient was pallid; blood pressure was significantly lower, and the repeat electrocardiogram during the discomfort now showed 3 mm horizontal ST segment depression in the precordial leads. I administered sublingual nitroglycerin. The discomfort ceased in 3 minutes, at which time the electrocardiogram returned to normal. The patient's postprandial discomfort was angina pectoris.

Clearly, most patients who have angina pectoris will have discomfort associated with physical exertion. Frequently, they may also have angina after eating. In this patient, however, *the anginal discomfort occurred only after eating, but did not occur with physical effort*. The clinician must be aware of this seemingly anomalous clinical occurrence.

Clinical vignette: An 87-year-old man complained of recurrent episodes of breathlessness and sweating that occurred only after eating. The symptoms would predictably start within 5 minutes of finishing his meal and always began while he was still seated at the table. The symptoms would spontaneously abate in 15 to 20 minutes.

While asymptomatic and having not eaten for several hours, his vital signs were normal. Physical examination did not reveal any pulmonary, cardiac, or intra-abdominal pathology.

I directed the patient to return to the office in a fasting state, but to bring a full meal with him. After a focused examination, I performed electrocardiography. Rhythm was normal sinus; non-specific ST-T segment abnormalities were evident. The patient then ate his food. Almost predictably, symptoms began after food ingestion. The heart rhythm was atrial flutter with a ventricular rate of 140/min.

Here is my point—when a patient's diagnosis is not clear, determine whether it is practicable to re-create the situation in which symptoms occur. Simple activities such as walking, food intake, or rising from the recumbent position cause patient symptoms. It is so logical, so easy, and so clinically rewarding to define the diagnosis by re-creating the situation.

Always Remember That Autoimmune Diseases Appear to Be Linked

The patient who has an autoimmune disorder is at increased risk to have another autoimmune disease.

Clinical vignette: One year ago, a 41-year-old woman had heat intolerance, profuse sweating, weakness, insomnia, and weight loss despite a robust appetite. Examination revealed tachycardia, increased pulse pressure, bounding pulses, lid lag, proximal muscle weakness, and exophthalmos. A diagnosis of Graves' disease was confirmed. The patient became euthyroid after long-term thionamide therapy.

However, a few months after the end of treatment, the patient again noted intermittent physical weakness, now with fatigable chewing, and intermittent diplopia. Ptosis, without papillary abnormality on the affected side, was noted. Clinical evaluation showed that the patient had myasthenia gravis.

Let us step back for a moment. What is the immune system?

Every day we hear of the immune system—what is thought to damage it, such as chronic stress, and what agents, often vitamin or herbal supplements, are marketed for strengthening immunity.

The basic function of the immune system is to protect humans from infectious organisms. The immune response is, primarily, the adaptation of the body to kill germs, also called microbes. The body's immune response to infection is to produce antibodies that attach to the invading germs and kill them.

Scientists have determined that it makes sense for the body to produce antibodies to a germ before that germ actually infects the body. Stimulating the body to produce these antibodies before actual infection prevents disease. This is preventive medicine at its best. So began the common practice of immunization.

But, in addition to reacting to disease-causing germs, the immune system also responds to noninfectious substances called antigens. Antigens are molecular substances within the body that excite the body as if the body is under attack. An autoimmune disease is one in which antibodies are produced that attack an antigen within the body of the host. The underlying reason why the body may produce antibodies against its own cellular antigens has not yet been determined.

Examples of autoimmune diseases and their antibodies are as follows:

Graves' disease	Anti-thyroid stimulating
Hashimoto thyroiditis	Anti-thyroid peroxidase; anti-thyroglobulin
Systemic lupus erythematosus	Anti-nuclear; anti-Sm; anti-ds DNA
Rheumatoid arthritis	Rheumatoid factor
Myasthenia gravis	Anti-acetylcholine receptor
Autoimmune hepatitis	Anti-smooth muscle
Primary biliary cirrhosis	Anti-mitochondrial
Scleroderma	Anti-nuclear; anti-Scl70

So, the patient who has autoimmune hypothyroidism may develop pernicious anemia or adrenal insufficiency. Or the patient who has myasthenia gravis may develop Graves' disease.

Always Assess Cardiovascular Status in the Man Who Has Erectile Dysfunction

I pose what I believe are interesting questions:

Is erectile dysfunction (ED) the earliest sign of generalized atherosclerosis in a man? What is the endothelial dysfunction in the *coronary artery* of the male who has atherosclerotic heart disease? What is the endothelial dysfunction in the *penile* artery *of the healthy man who has ED?*

First, coronary heart disease and ED have an important clinical linkage. They are both associated with hypertension, diabetes mellitus, smoking, and low serum high-density lipoprotein (HDL) cholesterol concentration.

More significantly, the endothelial dysfunction in the coronary artery in atherosclerosis is the same endothelial dysfunction in the penile artery of the healthy male, namely, decreased nitric oxide production. In other words, healthy men with ED have the same chemical defect in the endothelium of the penile artery as occurs in the atherosclerotic coronary artery.

Therefore, ED may in many men be the initial manifestation of generalized atherosclerosis. It then makes good clinical sense that the man with ED should have a careful cardiovascular assessment.

Always Think: "Stroke + Fever = Endocarditis" (Till Proven Otherwise)

In a patient who presents with an acute cerebrovascular accident, it is imperative to record an accurate body temperature (and a "stat" erythrocyte sedimentation rate). If the patient has a fever, immediately think first that the patient has endocarditis. Echocardiography and blood cultures are essential diagnostic modalities to be performed.

A patient who has an acute thrombotic stroke, subarachnoid hemorrhage, bland (noninfected) cardiogenic embolus, or intracerebral hemorrhage will not be febrile at the time of onset of symptoms.

Please see Chapter 2, "The Most Important Word in Diagnosis: *And.*"

Always Check for Radial-Femoral Artery Pulse Lag

In a patient who has hypertension, *always* check one time to determine whether a radial-femoral artery pulse lag is present.

Coarctation of the aorta is an important, treatable cause of hypertension. In most cases, the congenital narrowing of the aorta occurs distal to the origin of the left subclavian artery. Therefore, the blood pressure will be high and equal in both arms and lower in the thighs. Much less commonly, the coarctation is proximal to the left subclavian artery. In these patients, blood pressure will be high only in the right arm. Interestingly, the diastolic blood pressure is the same proximal and distal to the coarctation.

All patients with coarctation will have a radial-femoral pulse lag. Two questions naturally arise. First, why do we check the radial and femoral pulses and not other pulses for pulse lag in coarctation? The answer is that the radial and femoral pulses *are the same distance* from the aortic valve. Thus, the pulse waves in each artery should be synchronous.

Every year, in the physical diagnosis course I smile when I observe an inchoate student checking the *carotid and femoral* arteries for pulse lag. It is amazing that the student may find the pulses to be synchronous even though the carotid pulse is 3 or 4 inches from the aortic valve and the femoral pulse in the adult may be more than 2 feet from the aortic valve!

The second question is, "Why is there a pulse lag in the patient who has coarctation?" The answer is anatomic. Blood flow that is obstructed in the stenotic aorta is shunted through collateral vessels, specifically, to the intercostal arteries, and then to the superior and inferior recurrent epigastric arteries, and finally to the leg. This takes time; thus, the femoral pulse is felt after the radial pulsation.

Always Consider Fall Risk

Always remember that older adults are at increased risk of falling. Therefore, be particularly careful when prescribing medications that may disturb the patient's equilibrium, clarity of thought, and standing blood pressure.

Falls in the older adult may result from chronic disease, such as Parkinson's disease, osteoarthritis of knees and hips, diabetes mellitus, lower extremity weakness, reduced visual acuity, loss of proprioception, and imbalance from vestibular dysfunction.

The clinician must be aware that many medications might further increase risk of falling. All classes of medication used in therapy of Parkinson's disease have adverse effects that include dizziness, confusion, and orthostatic hypotension. Examples of other medications that warrant close attention are benzodiazepams, diuretics, and nitrates.

Always Consider Osteoporosis

Primary osteoporosis is bone loss associated with aging. *Always* remember that 25% of postmenopausal women will have *secondary* osteoporosis, that is, osteoporosis due to another disease and not simply related to the aging process.

Clearly, the estrogen deficiency plays a central role in causation of postmenopausal osteoporosis. However, the clinician must not rush to judgment in ascribing the estrogen deficiency as the etiology of the low bone mass and disordered bone architecture characteristic of this disorder. There are many causes of secondary osteoporosis in women. These include the following:

- Glucocorticoid therapy (even in a dose as low as prednisone, 2.5 mg/day)
- Hypercortisolism of other etiology, for example, Cushing's disease, adrenal hyperplasia, or carcinoma
- Hyperthyroidism
- Inflammatory bowel disease (Crohn's disease and ulcerative colitis)
- Organ transplantation

- Cholestatic liver disease
- Pancreatic insufficiency
- Celiac disease
- Multiple myeloma

Secondary osteoporosis occurs in men as well as women.

Here are key clinical points that you should remember about secondary osteoporosis in both sexes:

- Significant osteoporosis may occur in the patient who has *subclinical hypercortisolism*. Patients with subclinical Cushing's disease may have significant bone loss when they do not exhibit the classic manifestations including round, plethoric facies, buffalo hump, and depressed purple striae. What are clues that the patient has subclinical Cushing's disease? Hypertension, glucose intolerance, and dyslipidemia.
- Celiac disease deserves special mention. Adult patients with celiac disease who are between the ages 30 and 40 years typically have mild gastrointestinal symptoms, such as bloating and mild diarrhea. Yet significant osteoporosis (and iron deficiency) is common in these patients.

Remember these clinical clues to the presence of secondary osteoporosis:

  a. All men
  b. Premenopausal women
  c. African American and Asian women (osteoporosis is less common in these groups)
  d. Patients who have hypertension, glucose intolerance, and dyslipidemia
  e. Patients with resting tachycardia
  f. Anemic patients who have elevated erythrocyte sedimentation rate

Although primary osteoporosis of aging is very common, always seek clinical clues to the presence of underlying disease causing secondary bone loss.

Always Talk About Each Issue

Always remember to advise the patient, "Let's talk about that one" when the patient appears to have multiple and seemingly confusing symptoms.

Clinical vignette: A 76-year-old man presents for evaluation of chest pain. The patient was well until 3 months ago when he began to experience chest pain when swinging a golf club. The discomfort, described as "sharp," is located in the right upper lateral chest and right shoulder. When not swinging the club, the patient has no pain. The patient notes that, at times, he has a "tightness" in the anterior chest that radiates to the left shoulder. This discomfort occurs when the patient becomes angry in heated argument. The discomfort may last 10 to 15 minutes and is associated with mild breathlessness. The patient adds that for the past 3 weeks he has awakened with "burning" in the sternal area associated with a bitter taste in his mouth.

Let us review the history: The patient has a chief complaint of chest pain. Yet he is, innocently, linking three different types of pain as if they were of common origin. First, he describes a *sharp pain*, then speaks of a *tightness*, and last, of a *burning* in his chest.

The clinical principle: When a patient has multiple complaints, guide the history and say to the patient, "You have mentioned sharp pain. Let's talk about that one." Obtain the details about this symptom, and then move to the second discomfort, tightness. "Let's talk about that one."

By following this precept, at the end of the history it will be clear that the patient has three different chest pains and three different diagnoses: tendonitis, angina pectoris, and gastroesophageal reflux.

Always Remember That the Most Powerful Medicine Is *Reassurance*

Clinical vignette: A 68-year-old man, affluent and highly respected in his New England community, presented to my office in follow-up of a myocardial infarction that he had suffered 2 months earlier. From a cardiac viewpoint, his cardiologist in the north was pleased with his progress. He was free of anginal discomfort. Activity, though still modestly limited, did not cause breathlessness. He felt no palpitation.

The patient was in obvious distress as he continued speaking. He was anxious; he had lost confidence; angst was a daily burden. A full palate of anxiolytic medications prescribed by a psychiatrist yielded only feelings of drowsiness. He would not return to a psychiatrist.

In my conversation with the patient, he spoke only of his apprehensions. He volunteered that, since the infarction, he would not allow his wife to leave his side. I was incredulous that he would insist his wife accompany him to the bathroom.

My examination showed a furrowed brow and anxious expression. Vital signs were normal. Detailed cardiopulmonary examination was normal save a soft apical S4 gallop indicative of myocardial scarring. At the end of examination, I told the patient, "I have a powerful medicine that will help you." Quizzically, the patient asked how I would have a medicine not prescribed by others.

I took out my prescription pad and wrote the medication and its dosage. I handed the patient the prescription. On the paper was written "REASSURANCE." I explained that this medicine would enable him to regain robust health.

A full measure of reassurance, prescribed with sincerity and honesty, enabled the patient to finally recover from his heart attack.

Always Remember That Reassurance Is Your Most Important Medicine

Never

Never Ascribe Clubbing to Chronic Obstructive Pulmonary Disease

If the patient with chronic obstructive pulmonary disease has clubbing, look for another cause, especially lung cancer. Clubbing occurs in primary and metastatic lung cancer, cyanotic congenital heart disease, endocarditis (only left-sided), bronchiectasis, lung abscess, idiopathic pulmonary fibrosis, Crohn's disease, and cirrhosis.

Please see Chapters 1 and 2 for a more complete discussion of clubbing.

Never Diagnose Heart Failure Based on Unilateral Left Pleural Effusion

Never make a diagnosis of heart failure in a patient based upon the presence of a *unilateral left* pleural effusion. In heart failure, it is common for the chest radiograph to demonstrate a *bilateral* pleural effusion or a *unilateral right* effusion. However, presence of a unilateral left effusion should suggest another etiology to the clinician.

There are many causes of a unilateral left pleural effusion. The clinician must consider intrathoracic inflammatory diseases of the pleura, primary or metastatic lung cancer, pulmonary embolism, intra-abdominal inflammatory disorders, such as abscess, acute pancreatitis or pseudocyst of the pancreas, and intra-abdominal and pelvic tumors, including Meig's tumor of the ovary.

Transudative pleural effusions occur in the absence of pleural disease. Transudative effusions are noted in heart failure, hypoalbuminemia (cirrhosis and nephrotic syndrome), hypothyroidism, and pulmonary embolism. *Exudative* effusions are related to pleural or lung inflammation, or movement of intra-abdominal fluid into the pleural space.

Please do not misinterpret what I am expressing. By no means are all bilateral effusions or unilateral right effusions caused by heart failure; however, they are consistent with heart failure. A unilateral left pleural effusion is not consistent with a heart failure diagnosis.

You must remember:
1. Do not consider heart failure as the etiology of a unilateral left pleural effusion.
2. In the patient who has a unilateral left pleural effusion, think of pulmonary infection, intrathoracic malignancy, intra-abdominal infection, and intra-abdominal malignancy.

Never Order a Blood Urea Nitrogen Test Without Ordering a Serum Creatinine Value

The blood urea nitrogen (BUN) serum creatinine ratio is important in medical diagnosis. The average BUN/creatinine ratio is 8:1. However, it is more important that you remember that the *upper limit of normal for the ratio is 20:1.* Clinically, an increased ratio is more significant than a normal ratio.

Remember this basic point of renal physiology: Urea is reabsorbed in the tubules of the nephron. The amount of urea that is reabsorbed is inversely related to renal blood flow and glomerular filtration rate. In other words, reduced renal blood flow with decreased urine production is associated with more urea moving from tubule into the bloodstream. Thus, the plasma BUN concentration increases.

In contrast, creatinine production from skeletal muscle is relatively constant and is not reabsorbed in the tubules. As a result, the BUN/creatinine ratio is increased in conditions associated with a decreased renal perfusion. Examples include systolic heart failure and hypovolemia. This is called prerenal azotemia.

Excessive diuresis is another common cause of prerenal azotemia. Decreased cardiac output with its associated decrease in tissue perfusion causes an increase in the BUN/creatinine ratio.

Further, decreased urine volume due to urinary obstruction, either from prostatic hyperplasia or *bilateral* ureteral obstruction, increases the ratio because the reduced urine volume related to obstruction also promotes tubular reabsorption of urea. This is postrenal azotemia.

In acute tubular necrosis of the kidney, as may occur secondary to sepsis, hemodynamic shock, uric acid nephropathy, or myoglobinuria, the ratio is typically normal.

Note that an increased BUN/creatinine ratio also occurs in disorders unrelated to the kidney. Gastrointestinal bleeding, even occult bleeding, increases the ratio through a different mechanism. The proteins in blood (globin and albumin) are absorbed from the gut into the bloodstream. The liver converts these proteins into urea, thus increasing BUN concentration while serum creatinine is unchanged. In any patient who has an increased ratio, *always check the stool for occult blood.* Other, nonrenal causes of an increased ratio include intake of medicines that interfere with protein anabolism (tetracyclines and corticosteroids) and patients who have decreased creatinine production due to chronic illness with loss of muscle mass.

Obversely, a *low* BUN/creatinine ratio is found in patients with severe liver disease because hepatic urea production is impaired.

Never Allow Patients with Kidney Disease to Ingest Oral Magnesium or Aluminum

Never allow the patient with severe chronic kidney disease (CKD) to take magnesium- or aluminum-containing oral preparations.

Over-the-counter antacids that contain magnesium and aluminum are popular, for example, Maalox and Mylanta. Magnesium intake in the CKD patient may cause the patient to have nausea, vomiting, and flushing. Hypermagnesemia may progress to cause bradycardia, hypotension, somnolence, and paralysis.

Decreased renal function increases the risk of aluminum accumulation that may produce an acute neurotoxicity manifested by mental status change, coma, and seizures. Chronic manifestations of aluminum toxicity include osteomalacia and an iron-resistant microcytic anemia.

Never Suppress an Escape Rhythm

In cardiology, *never* suppress an ectopic focus that represents an escape rhythm in the heart. To be specific, do not administer any medication that reduces the inherent ability of that focus to produce a heartbeat.

The normal pacemaker of the heart is the sinus node because it has the greatest automaticity, meaning that it normally discharges at the fastest rate of all cardiac tissues. If for any reason the sinus node discharge is suppressed, either temporarily or permanently, or its discharge is prevented from spreading through the heart, that is AV block, a secondary (or tertiary) pacemaker will take up its function. The lower pacemaker will be at a slower rate.

There is a definite gradient in the natural frequency of discharge among the lower pacemakers. In descending order of rate of automaticity (intrinsic depolarization rate), the sinus node is followed by AV nodal tissue, followed by automatic fibers in the ventricles.

When the pace-setting moves away from the sinus node, the rhythm is called an *ectopic rhythm*. When the sinus node does not control the heart rhythm and a subsidiary pacemaker has to take over, the rhythm is a *passive ectopic rhythm*. A passive ectopic rhythm is an escape rhythm. In contrast, if control of the heart rhythm results from increased activity of the subsidiary pacemaker, the rhythm is an *active ectopic rhythm*. Premature beats (atrial, junctional, or ventricular) are examples of active ectopic rhythm.

Under normal conditions, the subsidiary pacemakers are kept under control by the fact that the sinus node generates impulses (action potentials) at an inherently faster rate than the cardiac pacemaker tissues in the AV node and ventricles. These subsidiary or lower pacemakers play an important protective role when the primary pacemaker, the sinus node, does not fire at an adequate rate.

Let us examine a few examples of escape rhythm, that is, *passive ectopic rhythm*. If the sinus node slows markedly, or if there is a period of sinus arrest, an AV nodal impulse will control the heartbeat for one or several beats. These AV nodal beats represent an escape rhythm and are not to be suppressed.

In the patient who has third-degree AV block (complete heart block), none of the atrial impulses are conducted to the ventricles. In third-degree AV block, the heart is controlled by two pacemakers, the atria by the sinus node and the ventricles by a slow, idioventricular pacemaker. The slow idioventricular rhythm is an escape *passive ectopic rhythm* and is not to be suppressed. If that idioventricular pacemaker is suppressed by a medication that inhibits the spontaneous generation of a heartbeat, ventricular asystole and death results.

However, it is clinically appropriate to accelerate a higher pacemaker that will, physiologically, quiet the passive ectopic focus. Of course, an example is the use of a cardiac pacemaker in complete heart block. The electrical impulse rate of the pacemaker is faster than the intrinsic passive idioventricular rhythm. Thus, the ectopic focus no longer controls the ventricular heartbeat.

Never Prescribe Medication to a Patient with Pre-excitation Syndrome That Slows AV Conduction (Unless an Electrophysiologic Study Indicates That It Is Safe)

Any medication that slows AV conduction, for example, verapamil and dilti-azem, beta adrenergic blockers, and digoxin, promotes cardiac impulse conduction through the accessory bypass (Bundle of Kent) fibers from atria to ventricles rather than the impulses moving normally from atria through the AV node to the ventricles.

Conduction through accessory fibers promotes development of AF with very fast ventricular rates, often reaching 300/min. This tachycardia can provoke syncope. Even worse, the AF may degenerate into *ventricular fibrillation* and result in sudden cardiac death.

Please refer to Chapter 1, "Medical Brevities," for more information.

Never Interpret Serum Alkaline Phosphatase Alone

Never interpret a serum alkaline phosphatase (AP) value without consideration of the serum gamma glutamyl transpeptidase (GGTP) value.

Clinical vignette: An 81-year-old asymptomatic man has elevation of serum AP, but the serum GGTP and serum calcium concentration are normal. What is a likely diagnosis?

AP is found in liver and bone; in contrast, GGTP is in liver and biliary cells, but *not* bone. Therefore, in bone disorders, such as Paget's disease of bone or bone metastases, the serum AP is elevated, but the serum GGTP is normal. In contrast, patients who have disease of the liver, biliary tract, or pancreas have elevated levels of *both* AP and GGTP.

Never Order Large Amounts of New Medications

When a patient is to start a medication that he or she has never taken, and the patient must take the medicine for a prolonged period, *never* order a large quantity of that medication in the first prescription.

Clinical vignette: An 81-year-old man is diagnosed with systolic heart failure. Therapy is initiated with an angiotensin converting enzyme inhibitor (ACEI). The patient is given a prescription for 100 tablets. After taking the second dose, the patient develops angioneurotic edema, a life-threatening adverse effect. The ACEI is discontinued and the patient is left with 98 expensive pills sitting in the medicine cabinet, never to be taken.

Clinical vignette: A 72-year-old woman with long-standing hypertension now has AF. The clinician determines that prolonged therapy with a nondihydropyridine calcium channel blocker is appropriate therapy for control of blood pressure and the heart rate. The initial prescription is for 100 tablets. After a few days of therapy, the patient stops the medication because of an uncomfortable sensation of dizziness and headache. A residual collection of unused medicine reminds the patient of her needless expense.

Whenever I encounter a patient who requires prolonged therapy with a medication that is new for him or her, I *always* order a small number (or quantity) in the first prescription to determine whether the patient can tolerate the new medication. I can accomplish this in two ways. Occasionally, I give the patient two prescriptions for the new medicine, one for 15 pills, the second for 100.

Alternatively, I might give the first prescription for 100 tablets but direct the patient to obtain only 15 from the pharmacy. If the patient tolerates the medicine well, the patient can then return for the remaining 85 pills in the prescription. Of course, subsequent prescriptions are for a large quantity.

Never Forget That Diuretics May Cause a Significant Decrease in Cardiac Output

Clinical vignette: A 61-year-old obese man has a 2-week history of exertional dyspnea without associated anginal discomfort. Blood pressure is 160/90 mm Hg. Examination shows an apical lift, S4 gallop, and bibasilar crackles. A diagnosis of hypertension and diastolic heart failure is made. Therapy is initiated with counseling on calorie and sodium limitation; furosemide and potassium supplementation are prescribed. One week later, the patient returns. He has lost 4 pounds and says, "My breathing is much better. The shortness of breath is gone. But, now I have less energy."

What is the patient telling the clinician? The patient's chronology of symptoms, from initial dyspnea to his present fatigue, clearly describe the pathophysiology of his disorder. The presenting symptom of dyspnea is related to the hypertrophic left ventricle (LV) that is stiff (noncompliant). The stiff LV causes left atrial mean pressure to become elevated. In turn, the elevated left atrial pressure is transmitted back to the pulmonary capillaries. The lungs become stiff from interstitial pulmonary edema and the patient is breathless.

With diuresis related to furosemide administration, the circulating blood volume decreases. This reduces intracardiac filling pressure and, as a result, there is decreased LV filling during diastole, that is, decreased preload. Decreased preload causes a reduction in LV cardiac output. The symptom of decreased cardiac output is fatigue or weakness.

Here are important clinical points: Diuretics can cause a decrease in cardiac output in patients who have diastolic or systolic cardiac dysfunction. When the patient taking a diuretic has new-onset or worsening fatigue, consider the adverse effect of the medication on cardiac output, in addition to other factors, such as electrolyte imbalance. Second, decreased tissue perfusion from a diuretic-induced decrease in cardiac output causes an increase in BUN and increase in the BUN/serum creatinine ratio.

Never Allow Yourself to Slip Into Clinical "Ruts"

I was born and raised in a rural village of 300 inhabitants. Many of the unpaved paths around town had deep ruts that had been carved over many years. Of course, there is another meaning to the word *rut*, signifying a monotonous routine. Over the years, I have been chagrined when bright clinicians fall into what may be called clinical ruts. Here are some examples:

- Every patient started on nitroglycerin therapy is prescribed a dose of 1/150 grain (0.4 mg).
- Every patient started on furosemide therapy is directed to take 40 mg/day.
- All dementia is Alzheimer's disease.
- All patients with peripheral edema and dyspnea have heart failure.

Clinical vignette: An elderly man has exertional chest discomfort. A diagnosis of angina pectoris is made based upon history (remember, angina is a diagnosis by history). Nitroglycerin 1/150 grain is prescribed. The patient reports that the sublingual tablets "don't work."

The prescribed dosage may be wrong.

Please refer to Chapter 7, "The Smartest Answer to a Medical Question: 'It Depends'" for more information.

Clinical vignette: As a faculty member in the health profession, I am often visited by students who relate stories of family members who are suffering from illnesses that are puzzling to both the patient and treating clinician.

Several months ago, a student told me that her grandmother was dying of heart failure. I, of course, expressed regret. Quickly, the student continued that grandmother was laden with anasarca and that there was, specifically, no evidence of liver or kidney disease.

The case presentation ended with the statement that this was "a funny kind of heart failure because the chest X-ray is normal."

I gently inquired of other cardiac symptoms, of personal habits, of potential exposure to noxious agents that could cause pulmonary parenchymal disease. After the student assured me that these were not contributory to the present illness, I responded, "Please call your grandmother's physician and, in a most respectful way, ask if he has considered constrictive pericarditis as the diagnosis."

Four days later, pericardiectomy was performed. In short order, the "heart failure" disappeared.

The attending physician had slipped into the rut of considering fluid retention as representing heart failure without critically thinking of other potential diagnoses.

Clinical vignette: A 71-year-old woman exhibited the classic manifestations of dementia. Blood count and red blood cell indices were normal. A quick diagnosis of Alzheimer's disease was made. However, the patient's husband requested consultation with another physician. A serum vitamin B_{12} (cobalamin) concentration was borderline low, and a serum methymalonic acid concentration was elevated. A diagnosis of vitamin B_{12} deficiency was made; the patient's mental status improved markedly with parenteral vitamin administration.

What happened in this case? The first clinician fell into the rut of considering dementia to be Alzheimer's disease without critically thinking of other treatable conditions that cause cognitive impairment.

Dementia may be the result of neurologic, endocrine, hematologic, or psychiatric disease. In addition to Alzheimer's disease, chronic alcohol abuse, Huntington's chorea, Parkinson's disease, and normal pressure hydrocephalus are associated with dementia. Depression is a common cause of "pseudodementia." Hypothyroid patients often have memory loss and a depressed affect. Oral bismuth intake, in excessive quantity, may cause memory loss.

Of even greater importance is the fact that some of these illnesses that present as dementia are treatable diseases. The dementia of hypothyroidism and depression is certainly reversible. Mental impairment caused by vitamin B_{12} deficiency or normal pressure hydrocephalus is reversible if the condition is diagnosed at an early stage.

Please see Chapter 1, "Medical Brevities," for a more complete discussion.

Never Say "Chest Pain"

When determining whether a patient has angina pectoris, *never* use the term *chest pain.*

In the United States, the word *pain* is typically used when one experiences an intense somatic sensation. In contrast, patients who have angina pectoris describe a heaviness, or squeezing, or constriction, or a mild burning sensation. This feeling may be sensed, most commonly, in the anterior chest, but may involve one or both arms, neck and jaw, the posterior chest, and upper abdomen.

In my experience, *at least half of patients with clearly defined angina pectoris will respond "no" when asked whether they have chest pain.* Therefore, when determining whether a patient has symptomatic myocardial ischemia, ask about "discomfort"—never "chest pain."

Never Administer Verapamil in a Wide QRS Tachycardia

Never administer verapamil to a patient who has a wide QRS tachycardia—unless you are *absolutely* certain that the tachycardia is supraventricular with abnormal intraventricular conduction (aberrancy).

A wide QRS segment is defined as equal to or greater than 120 msec (0.12 sec).

Arguably, the analysis of a wide QRS tachycardia represents the most difficult task in electrocardiography. The exigent question: Is the rhythm ventricular tachycardia (VT) or is it supraventricular tachycardia (SVT) with aberrancy? Several disorders can be responsible for a wide QRS tachycardia. These include the following:

- VT in which the heartbeat originates in ventricular conducting tissue or myocardium
- SVT: AF, atrial flutter, or paroxysmal SVT with fixed (permanent) left or right bundle branch block
- SVT: AF, atrial flutter, or paroxysmal SVT with functional bundle branch block due to part of the His-Purkinje system being only partially excitable
- SVT: preexcitation syndrome (Wolff-Parkinson-White) with ventricular activation occurring over an anomalous AV connection (accessory pathways)
- SVT: the wide QRS results from medicines, such as procainamide, quinidine, flecainide, encainide, propafenone, and amiodarone
- SVT: the wide QRS results from electrolyte abnormality, particularly hyperkalemia

Nothwithstanding the electrocardiographic criteria that have been established, the distinction between VT and SVT with aberrancy remains difficult, because the initial treatment to terminate the arrhythmia, the subsequent management, and prognosis are very different. Arriving at the correct electrocardiographic interpretation is more than an intellectual exercise.

The clinical lesson here is *not* whether you can define the electrocardiographic pattern of the tachycardia. You can call for help. The cardinal lesson is that the clinician who is not sure of the origin of the tachycardia should not give verapamil to the patient with a wide QRS tachycardia. The clinician must be sure to obtain a "stat" serum potassium level.

Why the concern over verapamil in this setting? If the rhythm is VT, the verapamil can precipitate severe hypotension and ventricular fibrillation. Only if the clinician is sure that the rhythm is SVT with aberrant intraventricular conduction (*but not preexcitation syndrome*) can the verapamil be given either to abort the arrhythmia or to slow the ventricular rate by the medicine's effect of slowing AV conduction.

Never Start a New Medication When the Patient Is About to Go Out of Town

It seems to be a most frequent occurrence. A patient, about to leave the community for a significant period of time, has a new illness, requires a change in therapy for a chronic condition, or is to be started on a medication never taken by that patient. A few days later, the treating clinician receives an urgent call (usually in the middle of the night due to time zone differences) from the patient expressing frightfulness or distress related to an adverse drug reaction.

Therefore, I try very hard *never to start a new medication when the patient is leaving the community*. Obviously, there have been times when the patient's medical situation is exigent, and I have no choice but to start the new medication. However, if at all possible, I wait for the patient's return before starting the new medicine.

Never Fail to Inspect the Patient Carefully During the Physical Examination

In my judgment, the weakest segment of the physical examination is inspection. The clinician "looks" but does not "see."

> Clinical vignette: (This is an unforgettable case, because this is the very first patient that I encountered, nearly four decades ago in clinical practice.)

A 26-year-old man presented to me with a chief complaint of newly diagnosed hypertension. He stated that he had just been released from a local hospital in which he had undergone extensive testing. No cause for the hypertension had been found.

Upon my examination, it was immediately evident upon inspection that the patient had acromegaly. He exhibited the enlarged jaw, coarse facial features, and enlarged hands and feet that are typical of this endocrinopathy. I told the patient that his hypertension was caused by a pituitary gland disorder that I very strongly suspected.

The patient never returned to me for follow-up. He went back to the physician who had missed the diagnosis and, shortly thereafter, underwent excision of a pituitary adenoma.

Clinical vignette: A 58-year-old man presented as a new patient in my office and told me that he had recently moved to Florida. Two months earlier, in the Northeast, he had undergone coronary bypass surgery and now wished me to care for him.

The patient was free of cardiorespiratory symptoms, and the cardiac examination showed a vigorous heart. However, the striking element in his examination appeared during my initial inspection. The patient had no pubic or axillary hair! Deep tendon reflexes showed a delayed relaxation phase. The patient had hypopituitarism. Almost expectedly, the patient returned for further evaluation to his physician in the Northeast. A few days later he underwent resection of a pituitary tumor.

My new cardiac patient did return to see me, now taking adrenal and thyroid hormone medications.

No, not all my cardiac patients had endocrine disease.

Never fail to inspect the patient carefully. The body habitus may reveal truncal obesity and depressed abdominal striae that will explain the patient's hypertension or hyperglycemia. The splinter hemorrhages in the nail beds in a patient with perplexing and persistent low-grade fever point to the diagnosis of endocarditis; in the patient with muscle pain, the splinter hemorrhages lead to the diagnosis of trichinellosis.

The signs that the clinician can find upon inspection are legion and cannot be fully described here. The important lesson is that the clinician must carefully *look*, must carefully *inspect* the patient at each encounter.

Never Discontinue Prematurely the ACE Inhibitor or Receptor Blocker

Never automatically discontinue an ACEI or ARB solely because of a small increase in serum creatinine level.

ACEIs and ARBs are important medications in treatment of proteinuric kidney disease, both in controlling hypertension and in preventing progression of the renal disease. Further, they are valuable medications in treatment of systolic heart failure and essential hypertension.

Every clinician is aware that an increase in serum creatinine value may be a sign of bilateral renal artery stenosis. As a result, many patients in whom ACEI or ARB therapy is initiated will have therapy *inappropriately discontinued* when there is a slight, stable increase in serum creatinine concentration.

The clinician should be aware that patients who begin taking an ACEI or ARB, or who have a dose increase, will demonstrate an increase in serum creatinine value. An increase in serum creatinine value up to 30% is acceptable if the creatinine value stabilizes at the higher value and does not continue to increase.

By following this clinical precept, the clinician can allow many patients to continue their beneficial therapy with these medications. A final point: Remember that *hypovolemia* makes a patient more susceptible to an ACEI- or ARB-induced increase in serum creatinine concentration.

Never Fail to Measure Blood Pressure and Pulse Rate When Checking for Orthostatic Hypotension

The two most common causes of orthostatic hypotension (OH) are sympathetic (adrenergic) nervous system (SNS) impairment and hypovolemia.

In the normal person, assumption of the upright standing position causes an initial blood pressure drop as a result of gravity. The carotid baroreceptors sense the fall in pressure and transmit impulses to the hypothalamus that, in turn, activates the SNS. Activation results in an increase in heart rate, arteriolar vasoconstriction, and venous constriction—all in an effort to maintain an adequate standing blood pressure.

Sympathetic dysfunction (SNS disorder) simply means that this system is not working. When a patient with sympathetic dysfunction, most commonly the patient with diabetes mellitus and neuropathy, stands, the expected, initial decrease in blood pressure occurs. Sympathetic activation *does not occur*; as a result, there is no increase in heart rate; there is no arteriolar constriction; there is no venous constriction. The patient will, at best, be lightheaded

Table 5–2 Review of OH

	Standing
OH due to hypovolemia	Pressure falls; HR increases
OH due to SNS disorder	Pressure falls; HR does not increase

or, worse, may faint. The blood pressure falls without a compensatory increase in heart rate.

Other causes of OH resulting from adrenergic dysfunction include these:

- Parkinson's disease
- Pernicious anemia
- Shy Drager syndrome
- Tabes dorsalis

In contrast, patients who have OH related to hypovolemia have OH, but the sympathetic reflexes function. Therefore, these patients have an increased heart rate when they stand up.

Hypovolemia and OH occur as a result of the following conditions:

- Hemorrhage
- Excessive diuresis
- Adrenal insufficiency

Table 5–2 provides a review of OH.

Checking heart rate and measuring blood pressure are simple yet highly valuable maneuvers to differentiate between SNS dysfunction and hypovolemia as the cause of OH.

Chapter 6

Linkages

Memorizing is attempting to learn without thinking. At best, memorization is but fleeting. However, learning embraced by thinking leads to understanding. Understanding is permanent. In the profession of medicine, understanding enables the clinician to make an efficient and correct diagnosis and, ultimately, promotes a logical approach to therapy.

I have found that linkages help me to understand and to be more knowledgeable. The linkage has no fixed structure. The linkages are limited only by one's creativity. Here are examples of linkage structures that I have created to help me in patient care:

- Laboratory value to body organ to physiologic response
- Symptom to pathophysiology to clinical questions
- Symptom to pathophysiology to physical sign to diagnosis

I hope that the following linkages will be helpful to you and will encourage you to create your own clinically useful linkages.

Linkage 1: Acid–Base Balance

Here, the linkage is *laboratory value* to *body organ* to *physiologic response*.

The human body can survive only in a very limited hydrogen ion concentration in the extracellular space. The hydrogen ion concentration is expressed as pH of the arterial plasma. The body has several systems that are vital in modulating hydrogen ion concentration. These include the lungs, the kidneys, and the blood. Acid–base balance, then, is the sum of all systems working together to keep hydrogen concentration in a narrow range in the plasma and extracellular space. The normal pH in systemic arterial blood is 7.35–7.45.

The Henderson–Hasselbach equation is integral to understanding acid–base balance because it expresses the relationship between two organs influencing pH, the lungs and the kidneys. Unfortunately, the Henderson–Hasselbach equation appears arcane, even frightening, to many students:

$$pH = pK + log \frac{(HCO3)}{(H2CO3)}$$

There are two components in the equation that are not essential to an understanding of acid–base balance. Let us remove them: exclude pK, an arithmetic constant, and log, an arithmetic exponent.

The Henderson–Hasselbach equation now becomes:

$$pH = \frac{HCO3}{H2CO3}$$

Because carbonic acid, H2CO3, is dissolved carbon dioxide (CO_2), we can substitute Pco2 for the H2CO3 in the denominator. As a result, the final Henderson–Hasselbach equation becomes

$$pH = \frac{HCO3}{Pco2}$$

HCO3 is plasma bicarbonate; Pco2 is plasma carbon dioxide tension.

This is the equation to remember. In summary, pH simply relates to the ratio of HCO3 (bicarbonate) to Pco2 (carbon dioxide).

Now, the linkages:

- *HCO3* is linked to *metabolic* that links to *kidney* with a final linkage to "*slow.*"

  Remember: The term *metabolic* relates to plasma bicarbonate. A low pH is acidosis; low pH associated with a low bicarbonate concentration is *metabolic acidosis*. Conditions that are associated with low bicarbonate include the following:

  a. Lactic acidosis

  b. Diabetic ketoacidosis

  c. Renal insufficiency

  d. Ingestion of methanol, ethylene glycol, or excessive salicylate

  e. Diarrhea, with excessive bicarbonate loss in stool

  A high pH is alkalosis; a high pH associated with a high bicarbonate concentration is *metabolic alkalosis*. Conditions that are associated with high bicarbonate include the following:

  a. Vomiting or gastric suction

  b. Loop or thiazide diuretic therapy

- *Pco2* is linked to *respiratory* that links to *ventilation* that links to *lung* with a final linkage to "*fast.*"

  Remember: Pco2 relates *only* to alveolar ventilation. If hypoventilation occurs, Pco2 rises and the Henderson–Hasselbach equation indicates that pH is reduced. A low pH is acidosis; a low pH due to elevated Pco2 is hypoventilation-induced *respiratory acidosis.*

  Obversely, if hyperventilation occurs, Pco2 in the blood decreases. According to the equation, pH must increase. A high pH is alkalosis; a high pH due to a reduced Pco2 is hyperventilation-induced *respiratory alkalosis.*

Now, let us turn attention to the *fast* and *slow* designators. What do they mean?

Fast and *slow* refer to *compensatory efforts of the lungs or kidney* in response to acidosis or alkalosis. If the primary illness is in ventilation causing respiratory acidosis (high Pco2) or respiratory alkalosis (low Pco2), then the compensatory mechanism is via the kidney. But the kidney is slow, meaning that it takes 3 to 5 days for the kidney to retain or secrete bicarbonate in an effort to keep the pH close to normal.

Here are clinical vignettes to illustrate the "slow kidney":

Clinical vignette, Patient A: A 24-year-old man is brought to the emergency department after having taken heroin. He is comatose and the respiratory rate is 6/min. The patient is *hypoventilating.* The CO2 retention is *acute*, the arterial Pco_2 is very high, and the pH is low. The patient has respiratory acidosis.

In an effort to keep the pH normal, the kidney would retain HCO3. The Henderson–Hasselbach equation states that $pH = \dfrac{HCO3}{Pco2}$

If the kidney would retain bicarbonate, then the pH would return toward normal in this patient who has elevated Pco2 and respiratory acidosis. But the kidney's response is slow, taking a minimum of 3 days. Therefore, in this case, the kidney *has not had time* to retain bicarbonate. The plasma bicarbonate level is normal, but the pH of the arterial blood remains very low. The patient has *uncompensated respiratory acidosis* because the primary problem is ventilation.

Clinical vignette, Patient B: A 62-year-old man has chronic bronchitis with chronic respiratory insufficiency. His lung disease causes him to retain CO2. Thus, his arterial Pco2 is high. A high Pco2 reduces arterial pH. However, this is a *chronic* condition.

Returning to the equation, $pH = \dfrac{HCO3}{Pco2}$.

The patient has a high Pco2 from his chronic bronchitis. Because the CO2 retention is *chronic*, the kidney *has had time* to retain bicarbonate in a compensatory effort to bring the pH back to normal. Therefore, the plasma bicarbonate level is also high. This is called *compensated respiratory acidosis* because the primary disorder is in ventilation and the secondary response is renal. *The key point is that the kidney responds slowly (3 to 5 days) when there is a primary respiratory acid–base abnormality.*

Here is a clinical vignette that illustrates the "fast lung":

Clinical vignette, Patient C: A 34-year-old man with type 1 diabetes has a 2-day history of fever and productive cough. He is brought to the emergency department in a confused state. Blood sugar is 520 mg/dL. Ketonuria is present. Systemic arterial blood pH is 7.29.

The patient's primary acid–base problem is acidosis. The acidosis is associated with a low plasma bicarbonate. Again, referring to the equation, $pH = \dfrac{HCO3}{Pco2}$

The low bicarbonate related to the patient's diabetic ketoacidosis is characteristic of metabolic acidosis. However, the lungs' response to an acid–base imbalance is fast. Therefore, in an effort to bring the pH back toward normal, ventilation quickly increases to "blow off" CO2 and reduce Pco2. In the case of diabetic ketoacidosis, the increased rate and depth of ventilation is called Kussmaul breathing.

The key point is that the lung can start its compensation in seconds to a minute when there is a primary metabolic acid–base abnormality.

Two other interesting clinical points:

- Acid–base compensation is never complete or perfect. In other words, the compensation brings the pH back toward normal, but the body does not reach a normal pH value.
- In the case of metabolic acidosis, a compensatory increase in ventilation never causes dyspnea. Thus, the patient who has Kussmaul breathing in diabetic ketoacidosis is never short of breath.

You must remember:
1. The arterial pH must be maintained in a close range for the individual to be alive.
2. The arterial pH is based upon the relationship of plasma bicarbonate (HCO3) to carbon dioxide tension (Pco2).
3. Simplify the Henderson–Hasselbach equation to: $pH = \dfrac{HCO3}{Pco2}$
4. Metabolic disorder = HCO3 = kidney = slow response
5. Respiratory disorder = Pco2 = lung = fast response
6. A disorder that is primarily associated with ventilation, e.g., pneumonia, drug overdose, causes a respiratory acid-base disorder with a compensatory metabolic response.
7. A disorder that is primarily associated with renal disease, an endocrinopathy, or gastrointestinal disease causes a metabolic acid-base disorder with a compensatory respiratory response. Examples include severe vomiting or diarrhea; uncontrolled diabetes; and uremia.

Linkage 2: Ptosis

Here, the linkage is *symptom* to *clinical questions* to *pathophysiology* to *diagnosis*.

One of the features that makes the practice of medicine so fascinating, interesting—and, sometimes, damning—is the fact that a symptom may have so many unrelated etiologies. Think of weakness or cough or vomiting or ptosis, to name a few.

Ptosis is a perfect example, for drooping of the eyelid may be caused by the following conditions:

- Infectious meningitis
- Bronchogenic carcinoma
- Autoimmune disease
- Vasculopathy due to hypertension, diabetes mellitus, or dyslipidemia
- Congenital anomaly
- Cerebral aneurysm
- Neuropathy due to sarcoidosis
- Brain tumor
- Carotid artery dissection
- Birth injury

You can see how linkage enables the clinician to follow a sensible course to diagnosis.

I suggest that four questions, quickly answered on physical examination, can lead the clinician to the correct cause of ptosis:

- What is the degree of the ptosis? (How far does the lid fall over the eye?)
- What is the pupil size on the affected side compared to the side without ptosis (equal, larger, or smaller)?
- Are the extraocular muscle movements normal or abnormal on the affected side?
- Do the ptosis and extraocular muscle movements vary with time?

Now, let us turn to the pathophysiologic mechanisms that relate to ptosis:

- *Sympathetic nervous system dysfunction.* A lesion along the sympathetic pathway in the eye, neck, or head may cause ptosis. Sympathetic nerve fibers innervating the eye cause dilation of the pupil and elevation of the eyelid via contraction of the small Mueller muscle.

  Sympathetic fibers *do not innervate skeletal muscle*. Extraocular muscles are skeletal muscles. Therefore, sympathetic nerves are not responsible for eye movement. The clinical point: Diseases affecting the sympathetic fibers in the brain and neck can cause *mild ptosis* (less than 2 mm) and miosis (pupillary constriction). Extraocular movement is normal.

  Ptosis, miosis, in association with impaired sweating on the same side of the face, is called Horner's syndrome. Be aware: In full illumination it is very easy to miss Horner's syndrome because the ptosis is slight (< 2 mm) and pupillary dilation is minimal. Examine the patient in dim light; only then will the anisocoria be clearly evident.

  The most common cause of Horner's syndrome is bronchogenic carcinoma of the lung apex that invades the base of the neck and affects the sympathetic nerves. The patient may have associated axillary or arm pain.

  Additionally, Horner's syndrome may be caused by brain stem stroke or tumor, dissection of the carotid artery, and cluster headache. Two points: Horner's syndrome is common in cluster headache and is *transient*, lasting less than 2 hours. Second, any patient who has new-onset Horner's syndrome associated with facial or neck pain *must be presumed to have carotid artery dissection*.

- *Cranial nerve III (oculomotor nerve) palsy.* The oculomotor nerve has two components, *motor* and *parasympathetic*. The motor fibers cause skeletal muscle contraction and, therefore, elevate the lid and effect most extraocular movements. The parasympathetic fibers cause papillary constriction. A small anatomic fact is important to remember: The parasympathetic fibers course along the outside of the cranial nerve. This has important clinical significance to be explained later.

An aneurysm of the posterior Circle of Willis, tumor of the sella turcica, meningitis, and head trauma can all cause paralysis of the oculomotor nerve. A patient with cranial nerve III palsy demonstrates *marked* ptosis, lateral deviation of the eye, abnormal eye movements, and a dilated pupil on the affected side. The affected pupil does not respond normally to direct light or accommodation.

What is the patient's complaint when the extraocular muscle movements are not normal? The patient has *diplopia when both eyes are open* because there is misalignment of the two eyes.

Now, back to the anatomic fact that parasympathetic fibers run on the outside of cranial nerve III. There are three conditions, diabetes mellitus, hypertension, and dyslipidemia, that may cause infarction of the *central portion* of the nerve. Here is the key point: These disorders cause cranial nerve III palsy manifest by ptosis and abnormal eye movements, but in 80% of cases the pupil size on the affected side is normal. Why does the pupil size remain normal? The answer is that the parasympathetic fibers on the outside of the nerve are not damaged by the vasculopathy involving the central portion of the nerve. Another important clinical point: diabetic third nerve palsy is often associated with periorbital pain.

- *Autoimmune disease*. Myasthenia gravis (MG) is associated with the presence of serum anti-acetylcholine receptor antibodies. These antibodies block neuromuscular transmission to *skeletal* muscles. The antibodies do not affect smooth muscle cells. MG affects the skeletal muscle in the eyelid and extraocular muscles, resulting in marked ptosis and abnormal eye movements. Pupil size is *not related to skeletal muscle*; rather, pupil size is related to sympathetic and parasympathetic innervation. The MG patient, then, has normal pupil size on the affected side.

  Here are the key clinical points in MG:

  ○ Pupil size is never affected.

  ○ MG is a systemic disease affecting all skeletal muscles. It is common for the patient to have weakness of arms and legs, even difficulty in chewing and talking.

  ○ Muscle weakness, including eyelid and extraocular muscles, is *variable during the day*. Weakness is typically worse at day's end. Upon arising after sleep, muscle strength may be normal or nearly normal.

Remember: In MG, ptosis and eye muscle movement abnormalities may vary during the day, but pupil size is always normal.

Using patient vignettes, let us review the linkage relating to ptosis. Again, the questions are as follows:

- What is the degree of ptosis?
- Are the eye muscle movements normal or abnormal?
- What is the pupil size on the affected side?
- Does the ptosis vary with time?

Clinical vignette, Patient A: An adult nondiabetic patient awakens with diplopia without associated eye pain. Examination shows marked ptosis, lateral deviation of the eye, and a dilated pupil. The patient has cranial nerve III palsy. Think of cerebral aneurysm or brain tumor as the underlying cause.

Clinical vignette, Patient B: An adult patient has the sudden onset of diplopia. Examination shows marked ptosis, lateral deviation of the eye, but *normal pupil size* on the affected side. The patient has cranial nerve III palsy but with normal pupil size. Think first of diabetes mellitus, and then hypertension or dyslipidemia as the underlying cause.

Clinical vignette, Patient C: A patient has marked ptosis and abnormal eye movements, but pupil size is normal. The ptosis and eye movement abnormalities vary with time. The primary underlying diagnosis is MG.

Clinical vignette, Patient D: A heavy smoker has an apical mass defined on chest radiography. Examination shows minimal ptosis, normal eye movements, and a constricted pupil on the affected side. The ipsilateral face is dry compared to the opposite side. The diagnosis is Horner's syndrome due to bronchogenic carcinoma.

Clinical vignette, Patient E: A 40-year-old woman who has had a dry cough for 1 month now has the sudden onset of diplopia. Examination shows marked ptosis, dilated pupil, and abnormal eye movements. Chest radiography shows bilateral hilar node enlargement. Diagnosis is cranial nerve III palsy secondary to sarcoidosis.

Sarcoid granulomas may invade any nerve to cause neurologic dysfunction. In fact, 50% of patients with sarcoidosis have Bell's palsy, a peripheral seventh cranial nerve impairment. The Bell's palsy may be unilateral or bilateral, simultaneous or sequential.

> **Clinical vignette, Patient F:** A 77-year-old woman has the sudden onset of diplopia. For 2 weeks, she has had right-sided headaches associated with scalp tenderness when brushing her hair. Examination shows cranial nerve III palsy. Erythrocyte sedimentation rate is 92 mm/hr. The diagnosis is giant cell arteritis.

A final note on ptosis: Congenital ptosis is *not* associated with a pupillary or an extraocular muscle abnormality.

You must remember:
1. Ptosis may be caused by "medical" or "surgical" (mass lesion) illness.
2. The cardinal questions to be answered on physical examination of the patient with ptosis are the following:
   a. What is the degree of ptosis?
   b. Are eye movements normal or abnormal?
   c. What is the pupil size on the affected (ptotic) side?
   d. Is the ptosis variable during the day?

Linkage 3: Peripheral Edema

Here, the linkage is *symptom* to *pathophysiology* to *clinical questions* to *diagnosis*.

Peripheral edema appears to be a ubiquitous clinical issue in medicine. It is addressed by the obstetrician, cardiologist, family practitioner, nephrologist, oncologist, gastroenterologist, and endocrinologist. Therefore, a linkage is essential to direct the clinician efficiently to the correct etiology.

Peripheral edema is palpable swelling resulting from increased volume of fluid in the interstitial space. Edema is not clinically apparent on physical examination until the interstitial volume has increased by at least 3 liters. In other words, the patient must gain at least 6 pounds in weight before the accumulated fluid produces noticeable edema.

In its most elementary form, edema may be produced either by an increased pressure in the capillary bed that *pushes* fluid from the vascular space into the interstitial space or by reduced oncotic pressure that *fails to hold* fluid in the vascular space, losing that fluid into the interstitium.

The pathophysiologic mechanisms causing peripheral edema include these:

- Increased capillary hydrostatic pressure
  - Heart failure
  - Expanded plasma volume
  - Deep venous obstruction
  - Pregnancy and premenstrual edema
- Low oncotic pressure
  - Hypoalbuminemia
- Increased capillary permeability
  - Injury to tissues
  - Medicines
- Lymphatic obstruction

Right heart failure and constrictive pericarditis produce edema because of the elevated inferior vena cava pressure extending into the capillary bed of the extremities. Additionally, in *chronic left* heart failure peripheral edema and increased capillary hydrostatic pressure result from heightened activity of the renin-angiotensin-aldosterone system promoting sodium and water retention. Salt and water retention that increases plasma volume promoting edema formation may be due to medication, for example, mineralocorticoids, estrogens, and non-aspirin, nonsteroidal anti-inflammatory drugs (NSAIDs). Nephritic syndrome, characterized by hypertension, hematuria, and mild proteinuria, results from glomerular damage that ultimately causes salt and water retention that produces edema. Nephritic syndrome may occur in post-streptococcal glomerulonephritis, infective endocarditis, lupus nephritis, immunoglobulin A nephropathy, and antiglomerular basement membrane disease. Deep vein thrombosis in an extremity causes a local increase in hydrostatic pressure and edema of that extremity.

Peripheral edema in pregnancy, even in uncomplicated pregnancy, is common. Increased hydrostatic pressure is caused by the increased plasma volume of pregnancy plus pressure of the gravid uterus on the inferior vena cava. Premenstrual edema may be caused by increased prostaglandin activity that promotes sodium and water retention.

Oncotic pressure holds fluid in the vascular space. Low oncotic pressure results from hypoalbuminemia. The low plasma albumin may be a result of urinary loss in nephrotic syndrome or, oppositely, of decreased hepatic albumin synthesis as is common in cirrhosis. The low oncotic pressure allows water to leak from the intravascular space into the interstitial space, producing palpable edema.

Increased capillary permeability allows water and albumin to move out of the capillary bed into the interstitial space, resulting in edema formation. This mechanism is responsible for edema formation in burns and in hypothyroidism. Medicines that increase permeability include human interleukin-2, thiazolidinedione agents such as pioglitazone or rosiglitazone, calcium channel blockers, and direct vasodilators such as minoxidil or diazoxide.

Lymphatic obstruction is most commonly a result of malignancy in which regional lymph nodes are infiltrated with tumor that inhibits local lymphatic drainage. In endemic areas, chronic filariasis due to nematode infection commonly causes peripheral edema resulting from lymphatic obstruction.

Here are the three clinical questions you must ask when evaluating the patient who has peripheral edema:

- Is the edema unilateral or bilateral?
- Is the jugular venous pressure (JVP) normal or elevated?
- Are the arms and face involved?

If the edema is unilateral, think of deep vein thrombosis or lymphatic obstruction caused by malignancy or infection.

Bilateral edema with *normal* JVP suggests hypoalbuminemia (hepatic or renal disease), hypothyroidism, and medication effect. Bilateral edema with *elevated* JVP is found in right heart failure, constrictive pericarditis, subacute pericardial tamponade, the rare restrictive cardiomyopathy, and SVC.

Note, however, that the bilateral edema in SVC syndrome *involves the arms*, not the feet and ankles. The arm swelling is often associated with facial edema and dilated superficial veins in the anterior chest. SVC syndrome is most commonly caused by malignancy (small cell carcinoma of the lung, non-Hodgkin's lymphoma), chest irradiation, or an indwelling central venous catheter.

Bilateral peripheral edema associated with *facial* edema is noted in nephrotic syndrome, nephritic syndrome, and hypothyroidism.

Periorbital Edema

A discussion of peripheral edema naturally leads to the subject of periorbital edema. The clinician may note periorbital edema in any patient who has facial edema. However, there are conditions that cause periorbital edema *without facial edema*. Causes of periorbital edema without facial edema include these:

- Allergy to aspirin and calcium channel blockers
- Sulfite allergy
- Trichinellosis

- Systemic lupus erythematosus
- Rosacea
- Hypothyroidism
- Angioneurotic edema
- Blepharitis

High sulfite concentrations are found in wine (red and white), dried fruit (excluding raisins and prunes), nonfrozen lemon and lime juice, molasses, and grape juice (white, pink, and red). Sulfite allergy, present in approximately 5% of asthmatics, can provoke *acute, severe asthma attacks*. Sulfite allergy seems to rarely cause acute bronchospasm in the patient who does not have asthma.

Angioneurotic edema is often related to medication intake, for example, angiotensin converting enzyme inhibitors (ACEIs), angiotensin receptor blockers, or nonaspirin, NSAIDs. Release of inflammatory mediators causes the rapid onset of edema that involves the lips, periorbital area, and, often, the laryngeal tissues. Angioneurotic edema may be life-threatening because of the danger of airway obstruction. If a patient is to develop angioneurotic edema from an ACEI, it *usually* occurs in the first few days after initiation of therapy. Rarely, however, the angioneurotic edema may occur the first time as long as 1 year after onset of ACEI therapy.

Trichinellosis resulting from nematode infection causes eosinophilia, muscle soreness, and splinter hemorrhages.

Rosacea is typically associated with flushing and telangiectasia. The eruptive component of the disease is associated with sebaceous gland growth leading to formation of pustules, cysts, papules, and nodules.

Using patient vignettes, let us review the linkage relating to peripheral edema.

Again, the clinical questions are as follows:

- Is the edema unilateral or bilateral?
- Is the JVP normal or elevated?
- Are the arms and face involved?

The Patient with Bilateral Edema

Clinical vignette, Patient A: A 66-year-old woman has *bilateral* peripheral edema, jaundice, spider angiomata on the chest, ascites, and transverse white bands in the nails except for a narrow band at the distal portion. JVP is normal. The diagnosis is cirrhosis; the edema is due to hypoalbuminemia from diminished hepatic albumin synthesis. The low albumin concentration results in low oncotic pressure. As a result, water moves from the vascular space (capillary bed) into the interstitial space, producing edema.

Clinical vignette, Patient B: A 47-year-old man has bilateral edema extending from the toes to the thighs. The arms and face are swollen. Urinalysis shows 4+ proteinuria. The JVP is normal. The diagnosis is nephrotic syndrome.

Clinical vignette, Patient C: A 61-year-old man has chronic bronchitis related to a long history of cigarette smoking. He now has a 1-week history of low-grade fever, increasing cough and sputum production, and worsening dyspnea. One day ago, he noted that his feet were puffy and his shoes were "tight." Examination shows central cyanosis, scattered pulmonary crackles, elevated JVP, and bilateral ankle edema. The diagnosis is cor pulmonale; the peripheral edema is due to the elevated jugular venous pressure that causes increased capillary hydrostatic pressure and fluid seepage from capillaries into the interstitial space.

Clinical vignette, Patient D: A 55-year-old man has a 1-month history of dry cough and 4-pound weight loss. Examination shows puffiness of his face, arms, and hands. The face is plethoric. JVP is elevated but without venous pulse waves. Chest radiography shows a right hilar mass. The diagnosis is SVC due to tumor, most likely small cell carcinoma of the lung or non-Hodgkin's lymphoma. Of course, biopsy is necessary to confirm the diagnosis.

Clinical vignette, Patient E: A 34-year-old man has an acute back sprain for which he has taken naproxen three times daily for one week. He now has puffiness of both feet. Examination shows blood pressure of 142/92 mm Hg, normal JVP, normal lung and cardiac examination, and 1+ edema of both feet. The diagnosis is edema and hypertension due to intake of a nonaspirin, nonsteroidal anti-inflammatory medication (NSAID). NSAIDs elevate blood pressure by inhibiting renal vasodilator prostaglandins. Further, NSAIDs increase sodium and water reabsorption in the kidney, which increases capillary hydrostatic pressure and produces bilateral edema.

Bilateral Edema Plus Facial Edema

Clinical vignette, Patient F: Two weeks after an upper respiratory infection, a 14-year-old girl has gross hematuria. Examination shows hypertension, a purpuric rash on both lower legs, bilateral ankle edema, and facial edema. Urinalysis shows red blood cells, red blood cell casts, and 1+ proteinuria. The diagnosis is nephritic syndrome related to Henoch–Schonlein purpura.

The Patient with Unilateral Edema

Clinical vignette, Patient G: A 49-year-old woman has a 2-day history of right calf tenderness and swelling of the right foot. Examination shows erythema and tenderness of the right calf, 1+ edema of the right foot, and a positive Homan's sign on the right. The diagnosis is deep vein thrombosis. The venous occlusion increases the capillary hydrostatic pressure distal to the occlusion, thus promoting edema only on that side.

Clinical vignette, Patient H: A 55-year-old man has had a surgical procedure for melanoma of the right arm. In addition to local excision, axillary nodes are excised. Postoperatively, the patient has chronic edema of the right arm. The diagnosis is lymphedema due to surgically induced lymphatic obstruction. *Chronic* lymphedema may become *nonpitting* in contrast to edema from increased capillary hydrostatic pressure that is always *pitting*.

Linkage 4: Dyspnea

In the following case, the linkage is *symptom* to *physical sign* to *anatomy* to *pathophysiology*.

Clinical vignette, Patient A: A 23-year-old man has a 2-week history of exertional dyspnea without associated cough, wheezing, or chest discomfort. Vital signs are normal. The patient is in normal sinus rhythm. The point of maximal impulse (PMI) is at the apex and an apical lift is felt. A 2/6 ejection murmur medial to the apex and apical S4 gallop are heard. Bibasilar crackles are noted.

Let's examine the linkage: The patient has dyspnea (the symptom). The apical lift (the sign) signifies left ventricular (LV) hypertrophy. Immediately, you are thinking that a hypertrophic left ventricle is a *stiff* (noncompliant) ventricle (the pathophysiology). For the left atrium to fill the left ventricle during ventricular diastole, left atrial (LA) pressure must increase. The increased LA pressure is transmitted backward through the pulmonary veins (there are no valves in pulmonary veins) into the pulmonary capillary bed. Interstitial edema develops and the patient has dyspnea. The S4 gallop signifies increased vigor of left atrial contraction as it tries to empty blood into the stiff, hypertrophic left ventricle. This is *diastolic heart failure* in a patient who has hypertrophic cardiomyopathy.

The cardinal element in diastolic heart failure is a stiff left ventricle.

The linkage in Patient A is as follows: LV hypertrophy → stiff left ventricle → increased LA pressure → increased pulmonary capillary pressure → interstitial lung edema → dyspnea.

Chronic Systolic Heart Failure That Eventually Becomes Combined Systolic and Diastolic Heart Failure

In the following case, the linkage is presented in a different pathway. Here the linkage is *symptom* to *sign* to *anatomy* to *pathophysiology* to a *new symptom* to n*ew pathophysiology.*

> **Clinical vignette, Patient B: A 73-year-old man has chronic mitral regurgitation, mitral valve regurgitation, and atrial fibrillation. The patient's chronic symptoms are tiredness and easy fatigability. Blood pressure is 90/70 mm Hg, pulse is 90/min/irregularly irregular, and respiratory rate is 17/min. Examination shows the apical impulse is in the sixth intercostal space in the anterior axillary line. A 2/6 apical holosystolic murmur and apical S3 gallop are heard. He has been treated medically with a loop diuretic, beta adrenergic blocker, and ACEI.**
>
> **The patient now tells the clinician that he has a *new symptom*. In addition to the generalized sense of weakness, he states that for the past 2 weeks he has exertional breathlessness (the new symptom).**

From a pathophysiologic basis, the patient is "telling" the clinician the linkage. First, the patient has been in *chronic systolic* heart failure manifest by a dilated left ventricle, reduced ejection fraction, and low cardiac output. The low cardiac output is the factor causing tiredness and easy fatigability. The patient had not been dyspneic in the past, because the mean LA pressure has been normal or nearly normal due to dilation of both left atrium and left ventricle.

Second, the onset of recent dyspnea indicates that the left ventricle has dilated as far as the myofibrils can stretch. The left ventricle cannot dilate any further; it is now *stiff* (the new pathophysiology). The stiff, noncompliant left ventricle now causes LA pressure to rise. The increased LA pressure, in turn, is transmitted back to the lungs and the patient has *cardiac dyspnea in addition to the tiredness and fatigability of chronic systolic failure*. The patient now has both systolic and diastolic heart failure.

Here is a review of the linkages in the patient who starts with chronic systolic heart failure and then exhibits combined systolic and diastolic heart failure: Initially, chronic mitral regurgitation → increased preload → dilated left ventricle and dilated left atrial → reduced contractile power → reduced ejection fraction → low cardiac output. This is systolic heart failure.

Then, the dilated left ventricle can stretch no further → increased LV stiffness → increased LA pressure → increased pulmonary venous pressure → increased pulmonary capillary pressure → dyspnea. This is diastolic heart failure superimposed on the chronic systolic heart failure.

The patient now has both systolic and diastolic heart failure.

Clinical vignette, Patient C: An 82-year-old man has stable angina pectoris. When walking too quickly, he experiences bilateral anterior chest pressure that radiates into his neck. The discomfort is associated with breathlessness. The patient stops walking, sits down, and places a nitroglycerin pill under his tongue. Within 2 minutes, the discomfort is gone and the breathlessness is gone.

In this case, the linkage is *pathophysiology* to *symptom* and, again, *pathophysiology* to *symptom*.

The patient has coronary heart disease with atheromatous narrowing of one or more coronary arteries. The increased oxygen demand placed upon the myocardium during walking produces myocardial ischemia. The symptom is angina pectoris. In addition, the myocardial ischemia causes the left ventricle to become *stiff*. As in the previous clinical vignettes, the stiff left ventricle causes an increase in LA pressure that is transmitted back to the lungs, causing pulmonary congestion and dyspnea.

Note the difference: In the patient with angina the LV stiffness occurs only during the period of myocardial ischemia and is, therefore, a *transient* stiffness. In the case of the patient with hypertrophic cardiomyopathy and the patient with mitral regurgitation and marked LV dilation, the stiffness is *permanent*.

The linkages are as follows:

- Coronary atherosclerotic narrowing of coronary artery → myocardial ischemia → angina pectoris
- Coronary atherosclerotic narrowing of coronary artery → myocardial ischemia → transiently stiff LV → increased LA pressure → dyspnea (transient diastolic heart failure)

Clinical vignette, Patient D: A 42-year-old woman has sarcoidosis complicated by diffuse pulmonary fibrosis and restrictive lung disease. Over a period of 2 weeks, the patient has a 7-pound weight gain associated with swelling of the feet and ankles. Blood pressure is 114/76 mm Hg, pulse is 116/min/regular, and respirations are 24/min. JVP is elevated. Scattered crackles are heard bilaterally on chest auscultation. The PMI is in the fourth intercostal space along the left sternal border. One plus edema of both feet and ankles is present.

What is the linkage of sarcoidosis to the elevation of JVP and peripheral edema?

The sarcoidosis is complicated by interstitial lung disease that, pathophysiologically, destroys the pulmonary vascular bed. The decreased vascular bed causes an increase in pulmonary vascular resistance that directly leads to the development of pulmonary arterial hypertension. The pulmonary hypertension causes the right ventricle to dilate and hypertrophy. As the pulmonary hypertension continues, the right ventricle fails and the patient slips into right heart failure characterized by elevated JVP and peripheral edema.

Note that the PMI in this patient with sarcoidosis is in the fourth intercostal space along the left sternal border. The PMI in this location is indicative of *right ventricular hypertrophy and dilation.*

The linkages are as follows: Interstitial lung disease (fibrosis) → destruction of pulmonary vascular bed → increased pulmonary vascular resistance → pulmonary hypertension → right ventricular hypertrophy and dilation → PMI in fourth intercostal space along left sternal border → right heart failure (cor pulmonale).

A brief review:

- Dyspnea with an apical lift as the PMI is *cardiac* dyspnea.
- Dyspnea with the PMI along the left sternal border is *pulmonary* dyspnea.
- Systolic heart failure is always associated with a dilated ventricle (increased preload), decreased contractile power, and low cardiac output.
- Diastolic heart failure is always associated with a stiff left ventricle.

Chapter 7

The Smartest Answer to a Medical Question: "It Depends"

Having been in the profession of medicine for 5 decades, it remains clear to me that technologic advances have not superseded or replaced what has been traditionally called the art of medicine.

Technology has not given us all the definitive, dogmatic answers that we seek when facing patients who have vexing clinical problems. Questions that arise when the clinician encounters these complex problems still have the same answer, "It depends." This chapter illustrates important medical questions for which the appropriate answer remains, "It depends."

It Depends 1: What Is the Proper Dose of Nitroglycerin?

It depends upon the blood pressure response to a sublingual dose of the tablet.

> Clinical vignette: It is very common for a referring physician to request consultation with a cardiologist for evaluation of a patient's complaint of chest discomfort. Not infrequently, the physician says, "The discomfort sounds like angina pectoris, but the patient did not respond to nitro. It must not be angina."

Of course, it is appropriate to question the accuracy of the diagnosis. Does the discomfort occur at times when myocardial oxygen demand is increased, for example, with walking, emotional upset, or sexual activity? Further, it is important to make sure that the nitroglycerin tablets are potent. (This should not be an issue for recently prescribed tablets.) Nitroglycerin tablets are heat and light sensitive. Tablets should be refrigerated, and patients should carry only a small number on their person. The tablets should be kept in a tightly sealed dark bottle. Patients should obtain a new bottle of nitroglycerin every 3–4 months.

Then, the important clinical point: Did the physician consider whether the dosage of nitroglycerin was the correct dosage? Nitroglycerin is a wonderful medicine if used properly—in proper dosage and in proper clinical settings.

The primary action of nitroglycerin is *venodilation*; only modest arterial and arteriolar dilation occurs. The venodilation results in a rapid decrease in venous return to the right atrium, thus reducing preload. As a result, the myocardial oxygen demand of the myocardium rapidly decreases. Anginal discomfort quickly ends.

The key clinical point: *Nitroglycerin is working properly if the systolic blood pressure in the sitting position decreases 10 mm Hg within 2 to 3 minutes after sublingual administration.* If the patient's dosage of nitroglycerin does not cause this hemodynamic response, the dosage is too low and the patient with angina pectoris will not have a beneficial response to the medication.

I suggest that clinicians counsel the patient with newly diagnosed angina pectoris on the following:

- Action of the medication.
- Its common side effects.
- Proper storage of the tablets.
- That nitroglycerin should be used, preferably, in the sitting position. If a tablet must be taken in the standing position, the patient should try to lean against another object, such as a parked car or tree.
- *That nitroglycerin does not work when taken in the recumbent position.*
- That the majority of patients who have angina pectoris can predict the activities most likely to provoke discomfort; therefore, the patient should sit down and place a tablet under the tongue 5–10 minutes before engaging in that activity. Examples of when prophylactic nitroglycerin should be taken include an expected vociferous business meeting, anticipated sexual activity, and the golfer approaching the first tee on the golf course.
- During an episode of angina pectoris, the patient should seek emergency aid if the anginal discomfort does not lessen at all within 5 minutes of taking the first tablet. However, while awaiting emergency assistance, if the discomfort continues, the patient may take 2 more doses at 5-minute intervals for a *total* of three sublingual nitroglycerin tablets over a 15-minute period.

Then, to determine the appropriate dose of nitroglycerin, the patient should undergo the following basic procedure:

1. With the patient in the sitting position, obtain three control blood pressure measurements.
2. Administer a dose of sublingual nitroglycerin.
3. Check blood pressure every 30 to 45 seconds for 3 minutes.
4. Determine systolic blood pressure response.

If the systolic pressure in the sitting position does not decrease 10 mm Hg, it is expected that the patient will not have a beneficial response to that dosage during an anginal attack. The patient requires a higher dose of nitroglycerin.

Obversely, if the systolic blood pressure while sitting drops more than 12 to 14 mm Hg, the dosage needs to be decreased because the patient is at risk of syncope, particularly if the medication is taken in the standing position.

You must remember:
1. The proper dosage of nitroglycerin in treating the patient with angina pectoris depends upon the blood pressure response to the medication.

It Depends 2: What Is the Significance of Atrial Premature Beats?

It depends on the *clinical setting* in which the atrial premature beats (APBs) occur.

> Clinical vignette, Patient A: A 27-year-old healthy man has an episode of paroxysmal atrial fibrillation of 8 hours duration. With electrical cardioversion the rhythm is reverted to normal sinus. One month later, while asymptomatic and anticoagulated, but not taking an anti-arrhythmic medication, ambulatory cardiac monitoring reveals frequent APBs.

In this patient without evidence of structural heart disease or intake of a provocative cardiac stimulant, APBs are a harbinger of recurrent paroxysmal atrial fibrillation. The clinician must consider reinstitution of anti-arrhythmic therapy. Electrophysiologic studies have shown that APBs, particularly in healthy persons, originate in the area of pulmonary veins and are a predictor of paroxysmal atrial fibrillation. Clearly, the anticoagulant therapy should be continued. If the ectopy cannot be medicinally controlled, the patient may be directed to undergo electrophysiologic study of the atrial ectopy.

Clinical vignette, Patient B: An 81-year-old man with coronary heart disease with remote myocardial infarction has a regularly scheduled office visit. The patient is asymptomatic. His unchanged medications include aspirin, a beta adrenergic blocker, and an HMG CoA reductase inhibitor (statin). The patient has gained 3 pounds since his last visit. Blood pressure is 110/72 mm Hg; pulse is 70/min with frequent premature beats. An electrocardiogram (ECG) shows normal sinus rhythm, APBs, and old anteroseptal myocardial infarction; there is no ECG evidence of myocardial ischemia. Review of previous ECG tracings indicates that the patient has not exhibited atrial ectopy in the past.

The key clinical point here is that APBs are often a sign of incipient heart failure, before the patient has heart failure symptoms and prior to appearance of peripheral edema or pulmonary crackles. However, the APBs may be accompanied by a new S4 gallop heard on cardiac auscultation. Note that the patient has gained 3 pounds since his previous visit, in this case a sign of early sodium and water retention related to heightened activity of the renin-angiotensin-aldosterone system.

By recognizing that the APBs relate to impaired cardiac function, the clinician can initiate heart failure therapy and, consequently, lessen the likelihood of an acute, emergent hospitalization.

Clinical vignette, Patient C: A 21-year-old woman has palpitations for 1 week. These are described as intermittent "thumps" in her left anterior chest. Examination shows a healthy-appearing but frightened woman. Vital signs are normal. Pulse shows occasional irregularity with premature beats. The heart size is normal; a midsystolic click and late apical systolic murmur are heard. An ECG shows frequent, single APBs.

APBs (and ventricular premature beats) are common in the patient who has mitral valve prolapse (MVP). The basis for the atrial ectopy (and the ventricular ectopy) is not defined. However, in the patient with MVP, initiation of beta adrenergic blocker therapy may reduce the frequency of APBs.

Clinical vignette, Patient D: A 20-year-old medical student, in the midst of preparing for final exams, is aware of an irregular beat in his chest. He is taking an over-the-counter caffeine preparation to stay awake for nighttime study.

Certain recognized cardiac stimulants provoke APBs. These include caffeine, alcohol, cocaine, and smoking. The atrial ectopy associated with caffeine intake and cocaine use is associated with increased adrenergic tone. The cardiovascular effects of cocaine are multiple and serious, including arrhythmia (paroxysmal supraventricular tachycardia and ventricular tachycardia), myocardial infarction (often, nonthrombotic), myocarditis, and dissection of the aorta.

Naturally, APBs induced by these agents are treated by counseling of the patient and discontinuation of the offending agent.

Occasionally, a patient who has systolic heart failure receives digoxin therapy in addition to the primary polypharmacy of beta adrenergic blocker, angiotensin converting enzyme inhibitor, and loop diuretic. Remember that APBs are an important early sign of digoxin toxicity.

In summary, APBs are nearly ubiquitous and are associated with many clinical situations, some entirely benign, others fraught with risk. The etiology and the significance of these ectopic beats clearly *depends* upon their setting.

You must remember:
1. APBs may be a harbinger of atrial fibrillation.
2. APBs may be a harbinger of heart failure.

It Depends 3: What Is the Proper Dose of a Diuretic in the Treatment of Heart Failure?

It depends on two clinical factors:

- Extracellular volume
- Renal function

Many years ago, in the early days of my cardiology practice, the national mortality rate for cardiogenic shock associated with acute myocardial infarction approached 70%. However, the mortality rate in those "cardiogenic shock" patients for whom I consulted was only 15%.

I was really good, according to my referring colleagues. Why were my cardiogenic shock patients faring so well?

Clinical vignette, Patient A (1970): An 81-year-old vigorous man without prior history of atherosclerotic disease has an acute myocardial infarction complicated by pulmonary edema. The patient was treated with nasal oxygen, intravenous morphine sulfate, and intravenous furosemide in a dose of 80 mg.

Six hours later, the patient was hypotensive and oliguric. I was asked to see the patient in consultation because the patient was in cardiogenic shock.

Clinical vignette, Patient B (1970): A 70-year-old man with known aortic valve stenosis was transported to the emergency department because of acute pulmonary edema. The patient was found to be in new atrial fibrillation with a ventricular rate of 140/min. The patient was treated with nasal oxygen, intravenous digoxin, and furosemide in a dose of 60 mg.

Five hours later, the ventricular rate had slowed to 116/min. However, the patient was now markedly hypotensive and oliguric. I was asked to see the patient in urgent consultation because of cardiogenic shock.

The clinical question: Were these patients in cardiogenic shock? Of course, no. In both cases, the patients had a *normal extracellular volume* (and normal circulating blood volume) at the time that they suffered their acute cardiac events, respectively, acute myocardial infarction and paroxysmal atrial fibrillation. The large doses of intravenous loop diuretic produced a vigorous diuresis followed by hypotension and oliguria *due to hypovolemia, not cardiogenic shock with its related feebleness in ventricular contractile power.*

My therapy for the cardiogenic shock in these patients? I carefully infused normal saline that brought the circulating blood volume back toward normal. In each case, there was a rapid and comforting rise in the patient's blood pressure, followed by an increase in urine volume.

Who are the patients with normal extracellular volume who are most likely to experience heart failure? Those patients with no prior history of heart disease who suddenly have an acute myocardial infarction, and those patients who suddenly have a tachyarrhythmia, either supraventricular or ventricular.

Patients who have left ventricular hypertrophy of any etiology are at particular risk for developing hypotension from diuretic therapy. The reduced circulating blood volume after diuresis can dramatically reduce left ventricular filling (preload), resulting in hypotension and a low cardiac output state.

In contrast, patients who have *increased extracellular volume*, that is, body water, are those with chronic heart failure with peripheral edema, cirrhosis with ascites and edema, and nephrotic syndrome. Patients who have these conditions have increased body water with *decreased renal perfusion*. Reduced renal perfusion means reduced diuretic delivery to the kidney. Additionally, these patients have heightened activity of the renin-angiotensin-aldosterone system, resulting in renal retention of sodium and water. The combination of decreased blood flow to the kidney and increased sodium and water reabsorption requires a *larger dose of diuretic* to effect diuresis.

Let us look even more closely at the patient who has cirrhosis with ascites. Although the extracellular fluid compartment is expanded, there is either an absolute or relative deficiency in intravascular volume. The cirrhotic with ascites, then, has a maldistribution of extracellular fluid. The ascites is not readily interchangeable with the intravascular space. When diuresis is induced with high doses of a loop diuretic, the fluid that is lost is coming from the intravascular space and it is not replaced by ascitic fluid moving into the circulation. Hypovolemia and prerenal azotemia result and can, ultimately, lead to hepatorenal syndrome.

Likewise, the patient with nephrotic syndrome is at risk of hypovolemia and hypotension from diuretics. This is because of low intravascular colloid osmotic pressure (oncotic pressure) related to hypoalbuminemia and maldistribution of extracellular fluid. The diuretic depletes the intravascular space. However, edema fluid cannot reenter the circulation at the same rate that the diuretic is reducing the intravascular volume.

Further, patients with *renal insufficiency* and increased extracellular volume require higher doses of a diuretic to produce an expected increase in urine volume. Multiple factors impair the diuretic response in a patient who has reduced renal function. These include renal perfusion, renal tubular reabsorption and secretion, and hormonal effects.

The bottom line: Patients who are in acute heart failure with a normal circulating blood volume should be treated with low doses of diuretics. Those who have an increased extracellular volume, that is, those with peripheral edema, and patients with impaired renal function require a higher dose of diuretic.

You must remember:
1. The clinician must consider the extracellular volume of the patient and the renal function before determining the dosage of a diuretic.

It Depends 4: Is Jugular (Central) Venous Pressure a Good Indicator of Hypovolemia?

It depends: Yes, the jugular venous pressure (JVP) is a good indicator of hypovolemia, but only *if the JVP is 0 mm*.

In clinical practice, an evaluation of extracellular volume is often important in the assessment of a patient. Increased extracellular volume is typically noted in patients who have chronic heart failure, nephrotic syndrome, and cirrhosis with portal hypertension and ascites.

Obversely, hypovolemia, that is, a reduced blood volume, is also commonly encountered in medical and surgical disciplines. Causes of hypovolemia include the following:

- Hemorrhage
  - Trauma
  - Rupture of aortic aneurysm
- Renal loss
  - Deficiency of mineralocorticoid (adrenal insufficiency)
  - Osmotic diuresis (uncontrolled diabetes mellitus)
  - Deficiency of antidiuretic hormone (diabetes insipidus)
  - Excessive diuretic effect
- Gastrointestinal loss
  - Hemorrhage
  - Vomiting
  - Diarrhea
  - External drainage
- Skin loss
  - Profuse sweating
  - Burns
- "Third spacing"
  - Crush injury
  - Intestinal obstruction
  - Pancreatitis
  - Major fractures

In all these conditions associated with hypovolemia, accurate assessment of circulating blood volume is essential to ensure proper management of the patient.

Therefore, the important clinical question is whether assessment of JVP is an accurate indicator of blood volume.

The Normal Body Response to Hypovolemia

What is the normal response of the body to *hypovolemia* of any etiology? The decreased circulating blood volume causes hypotension that is sensed by carotid baroreceptors. The baroreceptor sensors trigger a compensatory adrenergic response that includes acceleration of heart rate, increased ventricular contractility, and constriction of arterioles and veins.

The seminal role of the veins in maintaining an adequate circulating blood volume is often overlooked. Normally, about 70% of the blood in the body is in the venous circulation. The adrenergic compensatory venous constriction then increases venous return to the heart in an attempt to maintain preload, one of the cardinal determinants of ventricular function and cardiac output.

A most informative clinical test that was performed in healthy volunteers can explain why JVP is not an accurate indicator of circulating blood volume unless the JVP is 0. Healthy volunteers were subjected to worsening "hemorrhage" via application of lower body negative pressure. The negative pressure caused venous blood to pool in the veins of the lower abdomen, pelvis, and legs. As a result, circulating blood volume markedly decreased. In effect, the "hemorrhaging" patients exhibited the acute hemodynamic effects of hypovolemia.

When the circulating blood volume fell to a critical level, the volunteers fainted from the induced hypovolemia. At the time of fainting from "hemorrhage," the measured JVP was *normal* as a result of the intense compensatory venous constriction.

The clear conclusion is that JVP is a poor indicator of circulating blood volume. The clinician must use other signs, such as pulse rate, blood pressure, and particularly, blood pressure response to an upright position, as better indicators of hypovolemia.

You must remember:
1. JVP is a poor indicator of hypovolemia except when the JVP is 0 mm Hg.
2. JVP is always *elevated* in patients who are in right heart failure, have constrictive pericarditis, and pericardial tamponade.
3. JVP is typically normal in patients who have cirrhosis with ascites and those with nephrotic syndrome.

It Depends 5: What Are the Physical Examination Signs in Mitral Valve Regurgitation?

It depends on whether the mitral regurgitation (MR) is chronic or acute.

The signs of MR on cardiac exam depend on two factors, the volume of the left ventricular chamber and left atrial compliance. So infrequently do we speak of left atrial compliance, but it is of considerable importance, not only in physical examination, but also in the clinical status of the patient.

Chronic Mitral Regurgitation

The primary pathophysiologic impairment in MR is increased preload, the tension in the wall of the left ventricle (LV) at end-diastole. Preload, then, is the determinant of LV function that is related to ventricular volume. The increased preload causes the LV to become compliant and dilated. The apical impulse, then, is displaced to the left and downward on chest palpation. The murmur of regurgitation is typically plateau and holosystolic in character. Early, the dilated LV has an increased stroke volume (related to the Frank-Starling law). Later in its course, the dilated LV loses its contractile power, leading, ultimately, to systolic heart failure characterized by decreased cardiac output, reduced ejection fraction, and the symptom of fatigue.

As the vigor of LV systolic contraction lessens, the holosystolic murmur may decrease in intensity.

In chronic MR, the dilated LV fills rapidly during ventricular diastole and, thus, an S3 gallop (protodiastolic gallop) is typically heard.

Further, chronic MR causes the left atrial walls to become compliant and, resultantly, the left atrial volume increases. The left atrium (LA) is always dilated in chronic MR. This is a very important clinical factor because the compliant, dilated LA is responsible for the left atrial pressure to be normal or near-normal. With a normal mean left atrial pressure, the patient is not dyspneic. The patient may, however, suffer from fatigue resulting from the low cardiac output that occurs in systolic heart failure associated with chronic MR. Additionally, the dilated LA is an anatomic substrate for the onset of atrial fibrillation, which is very common in chronic MR.

In summary, the physical signs of chronic MR include the following:

- Apical impulse displaced to left and downward (dilated LV)
- Variable intensity of apical impulse (dependent upon LV contractile vigor)
- Apical S3 gallop
- Holosystolic murmur
- Irregularly irregular pulse (atrial fibrillation is common)

Causes of chronic MR include these:

- Mitral annulus calcification (common in the elderly patient)
- Ischemic heart disease (the associated LV remodeling leads to displacement of papillary muscles that, in turn, restricts closure of the mitral leaflets during systole)
- Left ventricular dilation of any etiology (LV dilation then causes dilation of the mitral annulus with appearance of MR; MR is common in dilated cardiomyopathy)

- Mitral valve prolapse
- Mitral valve distortion from healed endocarditis

Acute Mitral Regurgitation

Acute MR is rapid in onset, dramatic in clinical presentation, and life-threatening. In the setting of acute MR, the LV and LA do not have time to phys-iologically adapt. In other words, these chambers do not have time to dilate because they are noncompliant. The LV contracts vigorously in response to the sudden increase in left ventricular volume. Because the left atrial walls are non-compliant, there is an abrupt elevation in mean left atrial pressure. This sudden elevation in left atrial pressure is transmitted back into the pulmonary circula-tion. Thus, the patient who is catapulted into acute MR commonly presents with acute pulmonary edema.

The physical signs correlate with the sudden pathophysiologic cardiac abnormalities. The LV is normal in volume, so the apical impulse is not dis-placed. The noncompliant LA, faced with an increased volume of blood, has an elevated mean pressure that results in pulmonary edema. In the absence of left atrial dilation, the heart is in normal sinus rhythm and vigorous left atrial contraction produces an S4 gallop. The systolic murmur is dependent upon the generated pressure gradient between the LV and LA during ventricular contraction. A very high left atrial pressure reduces the gradient between left ventricular pressure and left atrial pressure; therefore, the mitral regurgitant murmur is softer and of shorter duration.

In summary, the physical signs of acute MR include the following:

- Normal LV volume (the apical impulse is not displaced but is dynamic)
- Systolic murmur that is variable in character (may be crescendo–decrescendo, that is, "diamond-shaped," or early systolic or midsystolic. Approximately 50% of patients with acute MR have *no heart murmur* noted on auscultation.)
- S4 gallop (because patient is typically in normal sinus rhythm)
- Pulmonary rales (because patient is typically in pulmonary edema)

Causes of acute MR in the patient who has a *native* mitral valve include these:

- Papillary muscle rupture (in acute myocardial infarction most often related to occlusion of posterior descending coronary artery; rupture may be secondary to chest trauma)

- Chordae tendineae rupture (due to endocarditis, trauma, or spontaneous)
- Flail mitral leaflet (due to acute infective endocarditis or MVP)

Causes of acute MR in the patient who has a *prosthetic* valve in the mitral position include these:

- Acute infective endocarditis eroding tissue valve
- Thrombosis or infection in a mechanical valve in the mitral position
- Regurgitation in the area of the mitral annulus (paravalvular) due to infection or suture rupture

---

You must remember:
1. The signs of acute MR are very different from the signs of chronic MR.
2. The clinician must know the different etiologies of acute and chronic MR.

It Depends 6: What Is the Duration of Anticoagulant Therapy in a Patient Who Has Deep Vein Thrombosis?

It depends on the underlying cause of the venous thrombosis.

If the patient has a *first episode of uncomplicated* deep vein thrombosis (DVT) resulting from a reversible condition, the DVT is treated initially with heparin, followed by warfarin for 3 to 6 months. Reversible conditions include the following:

- Pregnancy
- Trauma
- Hormone replacement therapy or tamoxifen
- Surgery
- Immobilization (extended bed rest; prolonged sitting during a long trip)

Indefinite warfarin therapy is indicated in those patients who have *recurrent DVT or a hypercoagulable state*. Conditions that cause a hypercoagulable state include Factor V Leiden mutation, antiphospholipid antibody syndrome, deficiency in protein C or S or antithrombin, and nephrotic syndrome.

In the patient who has DVT *complicated by pulmonary embolism*, duration of warfarin anticoagulation depends upon whether this is a first or recurrent embolus and whether an identifiable risk factor, reversible or irreversible, has been identified.

A few important clinical points:

- In 80% of cases, DVT is thought to arise in the veins of the calf. Half of these patients have no symptoms or physical signs. Others may show evidence of tenderness, overlying erythema, or a palpable venous cord.
- Oral contraceptive agents should not be given to women who smoke.
- Venous thrombosis in a woman who has experienced recurrent spontaneous abortions suggests antiphospholipid antibody syndrome.

It Depends 7: What Are the Electrocardiographic Findings in a Patient Who Has Angina Pectoris?

It depends on the following factors:

- Is the ECG performed while the patient is experiencing the anginal discomfort?
- Is the ECG performed during a provocative stress test?
- Is the ECG performed while the patient is in a resting, asymptomatic state?
- Does the patient have a prior history of myocardial infarction?

In my clinical years in practice, I have noted that the resting ECG is normal in at least half and, perhaps, up to three-quarters of patients with angina pectoris *when the tracing is performed at rest and the patient is free of anginal discomfort.*

During an episode of angina, the ECG becomes abnormal in approximately 60–75% of patients. Therefore, a normal ECG during chest discomfort does not exclude myocardial ischemia.

A common clinical vignette:

A middle-aged man comes to a medical office in a rather agitated mien and states, "I just want a cardiogram done on me. I don't need to see the doctor."

When briefly questioned by the nurse, he states that several days earlier he had an episode, while playing tennis, of "indigestion" lasting 5 to 10 minutes.

With the physician's acquiescence, an ECG is performed while the patient is asymptomatic. The patient is told that his cardiogram is normal. He departs the office convinced that he has no heart disease. The following day, back on the tennis court, the patient has severe chest pain and sustains an acute myocardial infarction.

Never give in to a patient's seemingly innocent request for an ECG to be performed. Never perform an ECG without a careful, focused history and cardiac examination in the patient who has had an episode of undefined chest discomfort.

Let us return to the original question: What are the ECG findings in a patient who has angina pectoris? If the patient with angina pectoris has left ventricular hypertrophy or ventricular dilatation, then the resting ECG tracing will be abnormal. If the patient has a history of previous myocardial infarction with pathologic Q waves, the tracing almost always will remain abnormal. However, an acute infarction in the past that was associated only with ST segment and T wave changes often reverts back to a normal ECG.

A note on electrocardiography: The subendocardial layer of the myocardium is most susceptible to insufficient perfusion, that is, ischemia. Electrocardiographically, the most specific sign of subendocardial ischemia (SEI) is horizontal ST segment depression or downward sloping (toward the end) of the ST segment. The T waves may become negative or remain positive.

T wave changes are unreliable indicators of myocardial ischemia. SEI may be associated with symmetrical T wave inversion, usually in association with ST segment depression. However, T wave inversion is less sensitive and less specific than horizontal ST segment depression in myocardial ischemia.

Nonspecific ST-T abnormalities (NSSTTA) relate to slight ST segment depression or T wave flattening (or inversion) that occurs without obvious cause. NSSTTA may occur in healthy persons who are in a state of acid–base imbalance (either acidosis or alkalosis), in persons shortly after eating, in those who are in a state of exaggerated sympathetic tone, or in those who have acute cardiovascular illnesses, such as pulmonary embolism or acute myocarditis. I have seen healthy patients who had a transiently abnormal ECG when the tracing was performed approximately 20 minutes after ingestion of a glass of orange juice.

It Depends 8: Does Carotid Artery Atherosclerosis Cause a Bruit?

It depends on blood flow and turbulence in the artery. It may appear incongruous, but here is a related question: Does airway obstruction causes wheezing?

Clinical vignette, Patient A: A 81-year-old woman has had two episodes of blurred vision in her right eye. Each has lasted a total of 4–5 minutes and is described as a "curtain slowly falling and then rising" in the visual field. Vital signs are normal. Both carotid pulses are 2+/4; a right carotid bruit is heard. Ophthalmoscopic examination shows moderate arteriovenous nicking.

Clinical vignette, Patient B: A 79-year-old man has a 1-hour history of left hemiplegia. In the emergency department, vital signs are normal. The right carotid pulse is not felt; the left carotid pulsation is 1+/4. No carotid bruits are heard. Cardiopulmonary examination is normal. Neurologic examination shows left hemiplegia, absent deep tendon reflexes, but an extensor left Babinski response.

Clinical vignette, Patient C: A 14-year-old boy has acute bronchitis that is worsening his underlying asthma. In the emergency department, initial examination shows the patient to be noncyanotic and without labored respirations. Diffuse wheezing is heard over the lung fields. The patient is treated with bronchodilator inhalations.

The patient initially improves, but 1 hour later his clinical status suddenly worsens. At this time, he is slightly cyanotic. Intercostal retractions are noted. No wheezing is heard.

A bruit is a sound produced by turbulent blood flow. Wheezes are musical sounds during expiration and, sometimes, during inspiration and result from localized narrowing within the bronchial tree. The narrowing is related both to bronchospasm and to inflammation in the bronchial tree. Wheezing breath sounds are dependent upon airflow. Patient C has worsening symptoms. *The disappearance of wheezing is a sign that the patient is clinically worse and that bronchial airflow is very low.*

Remember, first, that the intensity or amount of wheezing is not a good indicator of the degree of airway obstruction. Second, in the asthmatic patient who is improving, wheezing will *disappear* and in the asthmatic whose respiratory status is worsening, wheezing may *disappear.*

It goes both ways. The disappearance of wheezing may be desirable as airflow increases in a bronchial tree that earlier had been constricted and inflamed. The disappearance of wheezing, oppositely, may indicate that airflow is severely reduced from airway constriction and inflammation.

Patient A has amaurosis fugax. Although the origin of the blurred vision is small platelet and fibrin emboli arising in the carotid circulation, she still has adequate blood flow in the artery to cause sufficient turbulence to produce an audible bruit. In contrast, Patient B has a thrombotic stroke that is causing left hemiplegia. Occlusion of the internal carotid artery has so reduced blood flow that a bruit is not heard.

In summary, a carotid bruit alone is a *poor predictor of carotid artery stenosis* and subsequent stroke.

You must remember:
1. The presence of a bruit depends upon turbulent blood flow in the artery.
2. The presence of wheezing depends upon airflow in the bronchus.

It Depends 9: What Is the Significance of Hypotension?

It depends on circulating blood volume, systemic vascular resistance, myocardial function, and even the patient's body size.

Clinical vignette, Patient A: An 89-year-old woman who has enjoyed remarkably good health has a routine physical examination. Her only symptom is chronically dimmed vision in her eyes related to macular degeneration that now prevents her from driving her automobile. Examination shows a thin, petite woman who is alert and cheerful. Blood pressure is 90/70 mm Hg, pulse is 88/regular, and respirations are 19/min. Lung, heart, and neurologic examination is normal. The skin is warm and dry. Pulses are 2+/4 without bruits.

Clinical vignette, Patient B: A 78-year-old man has an acute anterior ST segment elevation myocardial infarction. In the emergency department, blood pressure is 78/52 mm Hg, pulse is 120/min/regular, and respirations are 28/min. The patient is cold and ashen. Peripheral cyanosis is evident despite nasal oxygen administration. Bibasilar pulmonary crackles and an apical S4 gallop are heard.

Clinical vignette, Patient C: A 66-year-old man with alcoholic cirrhosis has black stools for 3 hours. Blood pressure is 80/62 mm

Hg, pulse is 124/min/regular, and respirations are 24/min. The patient is icteric; palmar erythema and chest telangiectasia are noted. Stool is black and is markedly guiaic positive.

Clinical vignette, Patient D: An 82-year-old woman is transferred from a nursing home to the hospital because of fever and hypotension. Blood pressure is 78/56 mm Hg, pulse is 116/min/regular, and respirations are 24/min. Examination shows the patient to be warm, dry, and flushed. Lung, heart, and abdominal examination is normal. Right-sided costovertebral angle tenderness is elicited. Urinalysis shows marked pyuria with white blood cell casts.

Four patients, all with hypotension, yet with differing etiology, pathophysiology, and prognosis. Let's step back for a moment and consider the factors that relate to an individual's blood pressure level. They are as follows:

- Circulating blood volume
- Cardiac function, specifically, stroke volume, that is dependent upon
  - Preload
  - Afterload
  - Contractility
- Systemic vascular resistance

Hypotension is, obviously, characterized by low blood pressure. Clinically, hypotension should not be arbitrarily defined by a pressure level, a number. Rather, hypotension should be defined by its consequences, namely, impaired cerebral or renal function.

A low circulating blood volume, whether related to blood loss, increased vascular permeability, excessive diuresis, "third spacing" (ileus or severe pancreatitis), or dehydration results in decreased blood pressure levels. Patient B has low blood pressure due to blood loss, most likely from esophageal or gastric variceal bleeding.

A reduced left ventricular stroke volume may be related to abnormality in any of the three determinants of ventricular function, namely, preload, afterload, and contractility. Patient B, who is suffering from the acute myocardial infarction, has an acute decrease in myocardial contractility that reduces stroke volume and blood pressure. Any reduction in stroke volume results in lower blood pressure levels.

Gram-negative sepsis, as in Patient D, causes low blood pressure due to low systemic vascular resistance that is related to release of vasodilator mediators including nitric oxide and cytokines. Finally, sepsis increases vascular permeability, causing fluid to escape the vascular bed; this contributes further to hypotension by reduction in circulating blood volume. Sepsis most likely arises from urinary, gastrointestinal, and respiratory infection.

There are many healthy patients who, normally, have low blood pressure measurements.

You must remember:
1. Low blood pressure may be normal in certain patients, and very abnormal in others.
2. Cold, clammy skin indicates that the peripheral arteriolar vasculature is very constricted.
3. Warm, dry, flushed skin indicates that the peripheral arteriolar vasculature is dilated.

It Depends 10: Do Patients Who Have Infective Endocarditis Develop Clubbing?

It depends on the anatomic location of the endocardial/valvular infection and the duration of the infection.

Clubbing occurs only in patients who have *left-sided* endocarditis. Additionally, the infectious disease must be present for approximately 6 weeks before the clubbing is noted. Clearly, clubbing is not an early diagnostic sign in this disease.

Infective endocarditis is a disease with protean clinical components that can challenge the clinician's diagnostic acumen. The disease has four components, each serious:

- Cardiac valve destruction
- Distal embolization
- Metastatic infection secondary to bacteremia
- Immune complex disease with glomerulonephritis

In addition to endocarditis, clubbing occurs in the following conditions:

- Primary and metastatic lung cancer
- Lung abscess and bronchiectasis
- Cyanotic congenital heart disease
- Idiopathic pulmonary fibrosis
- Cystic fibrosis

- Hepatic cirrhosis
- Crohn's disease

Please see Chapter 1, "Medical Brevities," for more information.

> You must remember:
> 1. *Never* ascribe clubbing to chronic obstructive lung disease.

It Depends 11: In a Patient Who Has Coarctation of the Aorta, Is the Blood Pressure Equal in the Arms?

It depends on the anatomic location of the coarctation (narrowing) in the aorta.

In most patients with coarctation of the aorta, the anatomic locus of the arterial narrowing is *distal* to the origin of the left subclavian artery. Therefore, the systolic blood pressure is *high and equal in the arms* whereas systolic blood pressure is low in the legs. Diastolic blood pressure is equal in the arms and legs because it is, in large measure, dependent upon systemic vascular resistance. Radial-femoral artery pulse lag is a classic sign.

In the minority of patients with coarctation, the narrowing is *proximal* to the left subclavian artery. In these patients, the blood pressure is higher in the right arm than in the left arm. Rarely, the coarctation is *proximal to the origin of both subclavian arteries*. In these patients, the blood pressures in all extremities are equally decreased.

The clinician must remember these important linkages:

- Coarctation is commonly (~70%) associated with bicuspid aortic valve.
- Approximately 10% of coarctation patients have cerebral aneurysm.

What other condition is associated with cerebral aneurysm? Approximately 5% of patients who have inherited polycystic kidney disease (autosomal-dominant transmission) have cerebral aneurysm.

> You must remember:
> 1. Check for radial-femoral artery pulse lag in all patients who have hypertension.

Chapter 8

Clinical Potpourri

1. All Patients with Obstructive Sleep Apnea Snore, but Not All Patients Who Snore Have Sleep Apnea.

Snoring is a fixed feature of obstructive sleep apnea (OSA). These patients suffer from daytime sleepiness; further, they are at increased risk of systemic hypertension, pulmonary hypertension, and nocturnal arrhythmias, particularly bradycardia.

Remember that OSA occurs in children and may manifest as a behavioral disorder with inattention, impulsivity, even temper tantrums. It's not always attention-deficit-hyperactivity disorder. The etiology of OSA in children includes obesity and enlarged tonsils.

2. The Frequency of Attacks of Angina Pectoris Does Not Correlate with the Degree of Anatomic Stenosis in Coronary Atherosclerosis.

Patients with "mild" or infrequent angina attacks may have severe anatomic narrowing of coronary arteries. The rationale for performing provocative cardiac testing with nuclear or echocardiographic imaging is to assess objectively the extent of myocardium at ischemic risk.

3. Jaundice May Be Due to Elevation of Either Serum "Direct" (Conjugated) or "Indirect" (Unconjugated) Bilirubin Levels.

Hemolytic jaundice is characterized by unconjugated hyperbilirubinemia. The hemolysis may be *extravascular*, meaning that the red blood cell destruction occurs in the spleen, bone marrow, or liver. In contrast, the hemolysis may be *intravascular*, as occurs in sepsis, march hemoglobinuria, or hemolysis due to a defective prosthetic heart valve. Serum haptoglobin levels are reduced in both extravascular and intravascular hemolysis because haptoglobin binds to the free hemoglobin that is released during hemolysis.

Elevation of serum conjugated bilirubin levels occurs when hepatocytes are able to conjugate bilirubin, but there is obstruction to its outflow into the biliary tract. The bile then spills into the serum. Obstruction may be intracellular or extracellular, the latter often due to common bile duct pathology, for example, stone or tumor.

4. Iron Deficiency Is an Important Cause of Restless Legs Syndrome.

Restless legs syndrome is characterized by the following:

- An urge to move the legs, typically associated with an uncomfortable sensation in the legs.
- The urge to move and the discomfort occur at rest.
- Movement of the legs rapidly relieves the discomfort.
- Symptoms are worse at night.

Check the patient's hemoglobin and hematocrit, and also obtain a serum ferritin level in patients with restless legs syndrome.

Further, other patients may have fatigue and lethargy caused by iron deficiency manifest by depressed serum ferritin values. In these patients, the hemoglobin may still be in the normal range although the patient has distressing symptoms.

Iron deficiency may result from inadequate iron intake, malabsorption of iron, for example, in celiac disease and in intravascular hemolysis in which iron is lost in the urine in the form of hemoglobinuria or hemosiderinuria.

5. When Reviewing Laboratory Data on a Patient, Always Calculate the Blood Urea Nitrogen: Serum Creatinine Ratio.

The upper limit of normal of the ratio is 20:1. An increased ratio suggests one of the following conditions:

- Prerenal azotemia with reduced blood flow to the kidney, as occurs in systolic heart failure or hypovolemia.
- Postrenal azotemia with urinary obstruction in both ureters or, even, in benign prostatic hyperplasia.
- Gastrointestinal bleeding—always check the stool for occult blood in a patient with an increased blood urea nitrogen (BUN)/creatinine ratio.

6. The Patient Who Has Polycystic Ovary Syndrome Looks Like a Patient Who Has Cushing's Disease.

The woman with polycystic ovary syndrome typically has oligomenorrhea or amenorrhea, obesity, hirsutism, and increased risk of diabetes mellitus. Patients have increased serum levels of luteinizing hormone, estrogen, and androgen.

Patients with Cushing's disease also may be hirsute, obese (classically, truncal obesity), and have menstrual abnormalities and hyperglycemia.

It is easy to confuse the two conditions by appearance of the patient.

7. Diabetes Mellitus Is the Most Common Cause of Bilateral Loss of Knee Deep Tendon Reflexes.

The patient who has diabetic polyneuropathy has impaired pain, light touch, and temperature sensation in the distal extremities. Further, examination shows loss of vibratory sensation and proprioception in the toes. It is in these patients that deep tendon reflexes are lost.

8. Antibodies Are Present in the Serum of Patients Who Have Hypothyroidism Due to Hashimoto's Disease and in the Hyperthyroid Patient Who Has Graves' Disease.

Patients with Hashimoto's disease typically have antithyroid peroxidase antibodies and may have antithyroglobulin antibodies. Patients with Graves' disease have anti-thyroid stimulating hormone (anti-TSH) antibodies. Anti-TSH antibodies may be the only antibodies that *stimulate* the receptor, in this case, stimulating the thyroid gland to produce excess thyroid hormone.

Remember that patients who have one autoimmune disease are more likely to develop a second autoimmune disease. Therefore, myasthenia gravis and pernicious anemia are more likely to develop in patients who have Hashimoto's or Graves' disease.

9. Headaches and . . .

The older patient (usually over the age of 50 years) who has headache and a tender scalp has giant cell arteritis. This patient often has associated symptoms, such as jaw claudication (aching in jaw muscles while chewing), visual disturbance (amaurosis fugax), and polymyalgia rheumatic (vague aching in the shoulder and pelvic girdle). The erythrocyte sedimentation rate is typically greater than 75 mm/hr.

Headache and wet scalp and hair in a patient who has paroxysmal or sustained hypertension should raise suspicion of pheochromocytoma.

10. In Food Poisoning, Think of the Magic Numbers 40° and 150°F.

Food should be stored under a temperature of 40°F in an effort to inhibit bacterial growth and should be cooked to a temperature greater than 150°F to kill bacteria in food.

Why should cooked foods not be placed in the refrigerator while they are still hot? Because the hot food will raise the temperature in the refrigerator, thus allowing bacteria to multiply in other foods.

11. Examination of the Dehydrated Patient May Fool the Clinician; the Key Is in Understanding Osmotic Pressure.

Dehydration is not synonymous with hypovolemia. *Dehydration* means loss of plasma water without loss, or with relatively little loss, of solute (primarily sodium). This is typical in excessive sweating. In these patients, the loss of hypotonic sweat causes an increase in intravascular osmolality. As a result of the increased plasma osmolality, water moves out of the cells into the vascular space. The circulating blood volume is increased at the expense of intracellular dehydration.

The dehydrated patient complains of lightheadedness, weakness, and, perhaps, nausea. The mucous membranes are dry; the turgor is poor. But the vital signs may be normal because of the fact that the circulating blood volume is normal *at the expense of the intracellular space*. The vital signs, easily, could fool the clinician into thinking that there is minimal loss of body water.

In summary: Dehydration → increase in plasma osmolality → shift of water from intracellular space to intravascular space → "normalization" of circulating blood volume → normal vital signs.

Hypovolemia is loss of water and solute, as occurs in vomiting or diarrhea. The hypovolemia does not produce a significant increase in plasma osmolality. Water, then, does not move from cells to intravascular space.

Therefore, when the clinician examines a patient who has been repeatedly vomiting or has significant diarrhea, the circulating blood volume will be reduced. The patient may have resting tachycardia and hypotension; certainly, the presence of orthostatic hypotension reveals the extent of extracellular fluid loss.

12. Be Aware That the Patient Who Develops *Bilateral* Carpal Tunnel Syndrome Most Likely Has an Underlying Systemic Disease.

Carpal tunnel syndrome that involves both wrists over a period of a few months suggests the presence of one of the following conditions:

- Diabetes mellitus
- Hypothyroidism
- Chronic renal disease
- Acromegaly
- Rheumatoid arthritis
- Amyloidosis

13. Electrocardiography: Bundle Branch Blocks

Right bundle branch block (RBBB) may be a normal variant at birth and continuing through life. Acquired RBBB may represent hypertensive heart disease, idiopathic myocardial fibrosis, ischemic heart disease, infiltrative heart disease (sarcoidosis or amyloidosis), or inflammatory heart disease (myocarditis).

Left bundle branch block is always considered to be abnormal. The preceding cardiac disorders may cause this conduction defect.

14. Paradoxical Pulse: The Most Common Cause Is *Not* Pericardial Tamponade.

Paradoxical pulse (PP) is a classic sign found in the patient with pericardial tamponade. In the healthy person, systolic blood pressure during expiration is slightly higher (< 10 mm Hg) than during inspiration. PP is *not* a paradox; it is an exaggeration of normal. PP means that the systolic pressure during expiration is greater than 10 mm Hg higher than the systolic pressure during inspiration. The pathophysiology of PP is very complex.

Here is the technique to determine whether PP is present: With a sphygmomanometer in place, have the patient lie in a recumbent position and breathe *as normally as possible*. Inflate the cuff to a level above systolic pressure. Then, slowly bleed air from the cuff until blood pressure sounds are first heard. At this point, Karotkoff sounds are heard only during expiration because systolic pressure is lower during inspiration. Bleed more air from the system until Karotkoff sounds are heard throughout the respiratory cycle. The difference in systolic pressure at which only expiratory beats are heard and the pressure at which all sounds are heard is the size of the pulsus. Greater than 10 mm Hg difference is abnormal and is a paradoxical pulse.

The most common cause of PP is chronic obstructive lung disease (COLD). The pathophysiology is totally different from tamponade, but the physical sign is the same. The clinician is encouraged to measure blood pressure carefully in the patient with COLD to identify the presence of PP. This can make the determination much easier, at a later time, when the clinician evaluates a critically ill patient who is hypotensive with elevated jugular venous pressure due to tamponade.

15. Gynecomastia

In the older man who has gynecomastia, think of the following conditions:

- Cirrhosis
- Graves' disease

- Chronic renal failure with dialysis
- Medicines
  - Calcium channel blockers
  - H$_2$ receptors and proton pump inhibitors
  - Spironolactone
  - Digoxin

16. Arterial Blood Gas Determination

The arterial blood gas (ABG) values express arterial oxygen tension (PaO2), arterial carbon dioxide tension (PaCO2), and degree of acidity. From the data, the clinician can determine the arterial oxyhemoglobin saturation.

Therefore, there are three clinical indications to perform an ABG on a patient:

- When hypoventilation is suspected, that is, hypercarbia
- To determine oxygen tension (PaO2) and hemoglobin saturation
- To determine whether an acid–base imbalance exists

Hypoventilation leads to an increase in PaCO2 and reduction in PaO2. Hypoventilation occurs in chronic bronchitis, drug overdose, such as heroin overdose, and brain lesions involving the respiratory center.

Hypoxemia may be caused by five pathophysiologic mechanisms:

- Hypoventilation
  - An increase in alveolar carbon dioxide tension is associated with a decreased alveolar (and arterial blood) oxygen tension.
- Ventilation–perfusion (V/P) mismatch
  - V/P mismatch, either decreased alveolar ventilation compared to perfusion *or* increased capillary flow compared to alveolar ventilation, causes hypoxemia.
- Diffusion impairment
  - Inefficient transfer of oxygen from alveoli to capillaries results.
- Reduced inspired oxygen pressure
  - Breathing at high altitude without supplemental oxygen.
- Right to left shunting of blood
  - This could be considered an extreme example of V/P mismatch.
  - Anatomic shunts (pulmonary arteriovenous shunts).
  - Intracardiac right to left shunts.
  - Pulmonary disease (atelectasis, lobar pneumonia).

Central cyanosis is present if there is a significant degree of hypoxemia and the left ventricle is pumping increased quantities of unoxygenated blood. Cyanosis is apparent when the concentration of reduced hemoglobin is 4g/dL. Cyanosis appears when oxygen saturation is in the 75–85% range.

An important note: An abnormal hemoglobin, either genetic or acquired, can cause central cyanosis if the abnormal hemoglobin has a low affinity for oxygen. Methemoglobin is hemoglobin in which the heme is oxidized to the ferric state (in contrast to the normal ferrous state). Ferric heme is unable to bind to oxygen. Therefore, the patient who has methemoglobinemia is cyanotic.

Similarly, the person who suffers from cyanide poisoning and has cyanohemoglobin will be cyanotic because the abnormal hemoglobin is unable to transport oxygen.

Long-standing central cyanosis may lead to clubbing, but an abnormal hemoglobin does not cause this digital abnormality.

Peripheral cyanosis occurs when the left ventricle pumps a normal concentration of oxygenated blood, but blood flow is slow. The slow perfusion enables more oxygen to be extracted from the blood, causing cyanosis of distal structures, for example, fingers and toes. Slowing of blood flow occurs in the following conditions:

- Systolic heart failure
- Marked arteriolar constriction (may occur in some normal patients, usually female)
- Peripheral arterial disease

17. When Encountering a New Patient Who Has Hypertension, Always Check for Radial-Femoral Artery Pulse Lag.

Coarctation of the aorta is not rare. Further, remember that coarctation is frequently associated with a bicuspid aortic valve and, in approximately 5% of cases, is associated with cerebral aneurysm.

18. Butterfly Rash

Clinicians are clearly aware that a butterfly rash is the classic skin abnormality in the patient who has systemic lupus erythematosus. However, there are other disorders in which the rash has the same facial distribution. These disorders include the following:

- Sarcoidosis: the rash is called lupus pernio
- Acne rosacea
- Photoallergic or phototoxic drug eruptions
  - Sulfa, phenothiazines, tetracyclines, amiodarone, carbamazepine, furosemide, and tolbutamide may be offending medicines.

    Photoallergic reactions begin approximately 48 hours after exposure to the offending agent. The skin rash is not related to concentration of the medicine. Although the rash typically starts in sun-exposed areas, it may spread to other regions.

    Phototoxic reactions are related to concentration of the medicine and can occur in any person. The eruption is limited to sun-exposed areas.

19. Weakness

Physical weakness is a common symptom. Of course, the weakness may result from either upper motor neuron disease or disease of the peripheral nerves.

Upper motor neuron disease is characterized by weakness *plus* hyperreflexia, extensor plantar response, and disuse atrophy.

Peripheral nerve disease is characterized by weakness *plus* hypotonia, hyporeflexia, and muscle wasting.

This is the key clinical point: Muscle weakness without sensory symptoms or signs is rarely a result of peripheral nerve disease and should suggest neuromuscular disease (myasthenia gravis) or primary muscle disease (muscular dystrophy).

Index